Vegetarian Air Fryer Cooking Guide

A Comprehensive Collection of Quick and Easy Recipes for a Vegetarian Diet Using your Air Fryer

By Donna Thomson

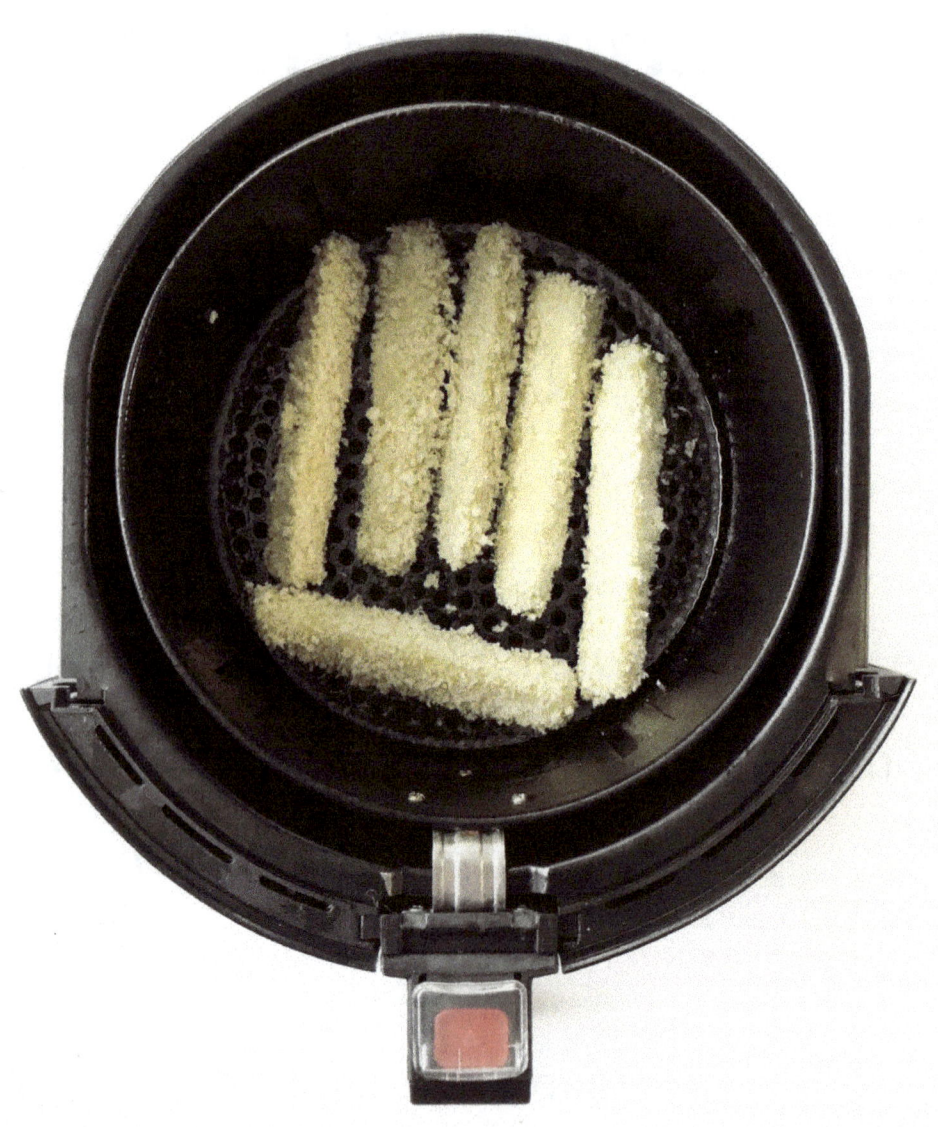

© Copyright 2021 - All rights reserved.

The content contained within this book may not be reproduced, duplicated or transmitted without direct written permission from the author or the publisher.

Under no circumstances will any blame or legal responsibility be held against the publisher, or author, for any damages, reparation, or monetary loss due to the information contained within this book. Either directly or indirectly.

Legal Notice:

This book is copyright protected. This book is only for personal use. You cannot amend, distribute, sell, use, quote or paraphrase any part, or the content within this book, without the consent of the author or publisher.

Disclaimer Notice:

Please note the information contained within this document is for educational and entertainment purposes only. All effort has been executed to present accurate, up to date, and reliable, complete information. No warranties of any kind are declared or implied. Readers acknowledge that the author is not engaging in the rendering of legal, financial, medical or professional advice. The content within this book has been derived from various sources. Please consult a licensed professional before attempting any techniques outlined in this book.

By reading this document, the reader agrees that under no circumstances is the author responsible for any losses, direct or indirect, which are incurred as a result of the use of information contained within this document, including, but not limited to, — errors, omissions, or inaccuracies.

Table of Contents

Brown Rice, Spinach 'n Tofu Frittata 10

Brussels sprouts with Balsamic Oil 12

Buttered Carrot-Zucchini with Mayo 14

Cauliflower Steak with Thick Sauce 16

Cheddar, Squash 'n Zucchini Casserole 19

Cheesy BBQ Tater Tot 21

Chives 'n Thyme Spiced Veggie Burger 24

Coconut Battered Cauliflower Bites 26

Creamy 'n Cheese Broccoli Bake 29

Creole Seasoned Vegetables 31

Crisped Baked Cheese Stuffed Chile Pepper 33

Crisped Noodle Salad Chinese Style 36

Crisped Tofu with Paprika 38

Crispy 'n Healthy Avocado Fingers 40

Crispy 'n Savory Spring Rolls 42

Crispy Asparagus Dipped in Paprika-Garlic Spice 44

Crispy Fry Green Tomatoes 46

Crispy Onion Seasoned with Paprika 'n Cajun 48

Crispy Vegetarian Ravioli 51

Crispy Veggie Tempura Style 53

Crispy Wings with Lemony Old Bay Spice 55

Curry 'n Coriander Spiced Bread Rolls 57

Easy Baked Root Veggies 59

Easy Fry Portobello Mushroom 60

Egg-Less Spinach Quiche 62

Fried Broccoli Recipe From India 64

Fried Chickpea-Fig on Arugula 65

Fried Falafel Recipe from the Middle East 68

Fried Tofu Recipe from Malaysia 70

Garlic 'n Basil Crackers 72

Garlic-Wine Flavored Vegetables 75

Grilled 'n Glazed Strawberries 77

Grilled 'n Spiced Tomatoes on Garden Salad 79

Grilled Drunken Mushrooms 82

Grilled Eggplant with Cumin-Paprika Spice 84

Grilled Olive-Tomato with Dill-Parsley Oil 86

Healthy Apple-licious Chips 89

Healthy Breakfast Casserole 90

Herby Veggie Cornish Pasties 92

Herby Zucchini 'n Eggplant Bake 94

Hollandaise Topped Grilled Asparagus 97

Italian Seasoned Easy Pasta Chips 99

Jackfruit-Cream Cheese Rangoon 100

Jalapeno Stuffed with Bacon 'n Cheeses 101

Layered Tortilla Bake 103

Loaded Brekky Hash Browns 105

Melted Cheese 'n Almonds on Tomato 107

Minty Green Beans with Shallots 109

Brown Rice, Spinach 'n Tofu Frittata

Serves: 4

Cooking Time: 55 minutes

Ingredients:

- ½ cup baby spinach, chopped /65G
- ½ cup kale, chopped /65G
- ½ onion, chopped
- ½ teaspoon turmeric /2.5G
- 1 ¾ cups brown rice, cooked /218G
- 1 flax egg (1 tablespoon or 15G flaxseed meal + 3 tablespoons or 45ML cold water)
- 1 package firm tofu
- 1 tablespoon organic olive oil /15ML
- 1 yellow pepper, chopped
- 2 tablespoons soy sauce /30ML
- 2 teaspoons arrowroot powder /10G
- 2 teaspoons Dijon mustard /10G
- 2/3 cup almond milk /167ML
- 3 big mushrooms, chopped
- 3 tablespoons nutritional yeast /45G
- 4 cloves garlic, crushed
- 4 spring onions, chopped
- a few basil leaves, chopped

Instructions:

1) Preheat the air fryer to 375° F or 191°C. Grease a skillet with oil.
2) To prepare the frittata crust mix the brown rice and flax egg together. Flatten the rice to the baking pan and a rice crust will be formed. Polish the crust with oil and cook for 10 minutes.
3) Heat extra virgin olive oil in another skillet over medium heat and sauté the garlic and onions for 2 minutes.
4) Add the pepper and mushroom and continue stirring for 3 minutes.
5) Add kale, spinach, spring onions, and basil while stirring. Scoop the content from the pan and set it aside.
6) Add the tofu, mustard, turmeric, soy sauce, nutritional yeast, vegan milk and arrowroot powder in a blender and blend to smooth. Pour the content in a mixing bowl, add sautéed vegetables and stir.
7) Pour the vegan frittata mixture into the rice crust and cook in the air fryer for 40 minutes.

Nutrition information:

- Calories per serving: 226
- Carbohydrates: 30.44g
- Protein: 10.69g
- Fat: 8.05g

Brussels sprouts with Balsamic Oil

Serves: 4

Cooking Time: 15

Ingredients:

- ¼ teaspoon salt /1.25G
- 1 tablespoon balsamic vinegar /15ML
- 2 cups Brussels sprouts, halved /260G
- 2 tablespoons essential olive oil /30ML

Instructions:

1) Put on the air fryer and preheat for 5 minutes.
2) Grab a bowl, put all the ingredients in it and mix well to coat the zucchini fries.
3) Place the bowl in the mid-air fryer basket.
4) Allow to cook at 350° F or 177°C for 15 minutes.

Nutrition information:

- Calories per serving: 82
- Carbohydrates: 4.6g
- Protein: 1.5g
- Fat: 6.8g

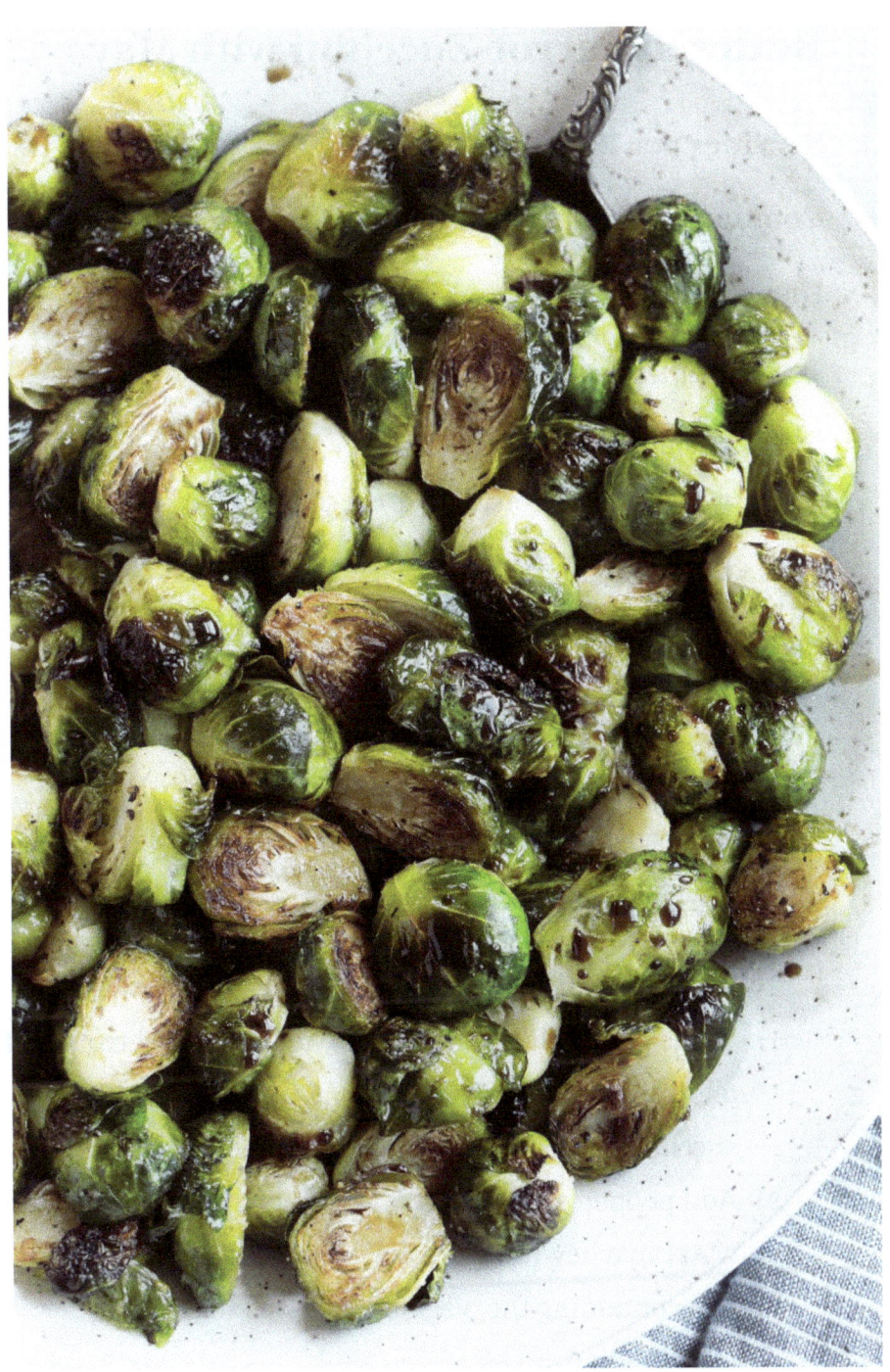

Buttered Carrot-Zucchini with Mayo

Servings per Recipe: 4

Cooking Time: 25 minutes

Ingredients:

- 1 tablespoon grated onion /15G
- 2 tablespoons butter, melted /30ML
- 1/2-pound carrots, sliced /225G
- 1-1/2 zucchinis, sliced
- 1/4 cup water /62.5ML
- 1/4 cup mayonnaise /62.5ML
- 1/4 teaspoon prepared horseradish /1.25G
- 1/4 teaspoon salt /1.25G
- 1/4 teaspoon ground black pepper /1.25G
- ==1/4 cup Italian bread crumbs /32.5G==

Instructions

1) Grease the baking pan lightly with oil. Add carrots and allow to cook at 360° F or 183°C for 8 minutes. Add zucchini and continue cooking for another 5 minutes.
2) Add pepper, salt, horseradish, onion, mayonnaise, and water in a bowl and mix well. Pour this content into the pan containing the veggies. Mix well to coat.

3) In another bowl mix melted butter and bread crumbs. Sprinkle over veggies.
4) Cook for 10 at 390° F or 199°C until the toppings are lightly browned.
5) Serve and enjoy.

Nutrition Information:

- Calories per Serving: 223
- Carbs: 13.8g
- Protein: 2.7g
- Fat: 17.4g

Cauliflower Steak with Thick Sauce

Serves: 2

Cooking Time: 15

Ingredients:

- ¼ cup almond milk /62.5ML
- ¼ teaspoon vegetable stock powder /1.25G
- 1 cauliflower, sliced into two
- 1 tablespoon olive oil /15ML
- 2 tablespoons onion, chopped /30G
- Salt and pepper to taste

Instructions:

1) Brine or soak cauliflower in salted water for around 2 hours while preheating the air fryer to 400° F or 205°C.
2) Rinse the salt off the cauliflower, place in the air fryer and cook for 15 minutes.
3) Heat oil in a frying pan over medium heat. Sauté the onions and stir until tender. Sprinkle vegetable stock powder and milk.
4) Allow to boil and reduce heat to low.
5) Allow the sauce to cook well and season with salt and pepper.
6) Serve cauliflower steak on a plate and pour the sauce on it.

Nutrition information:

- Calories per serving: 91
- Carbohydrates: 6.58 g
- Protein: 1.02g
- Fat: 7.22g

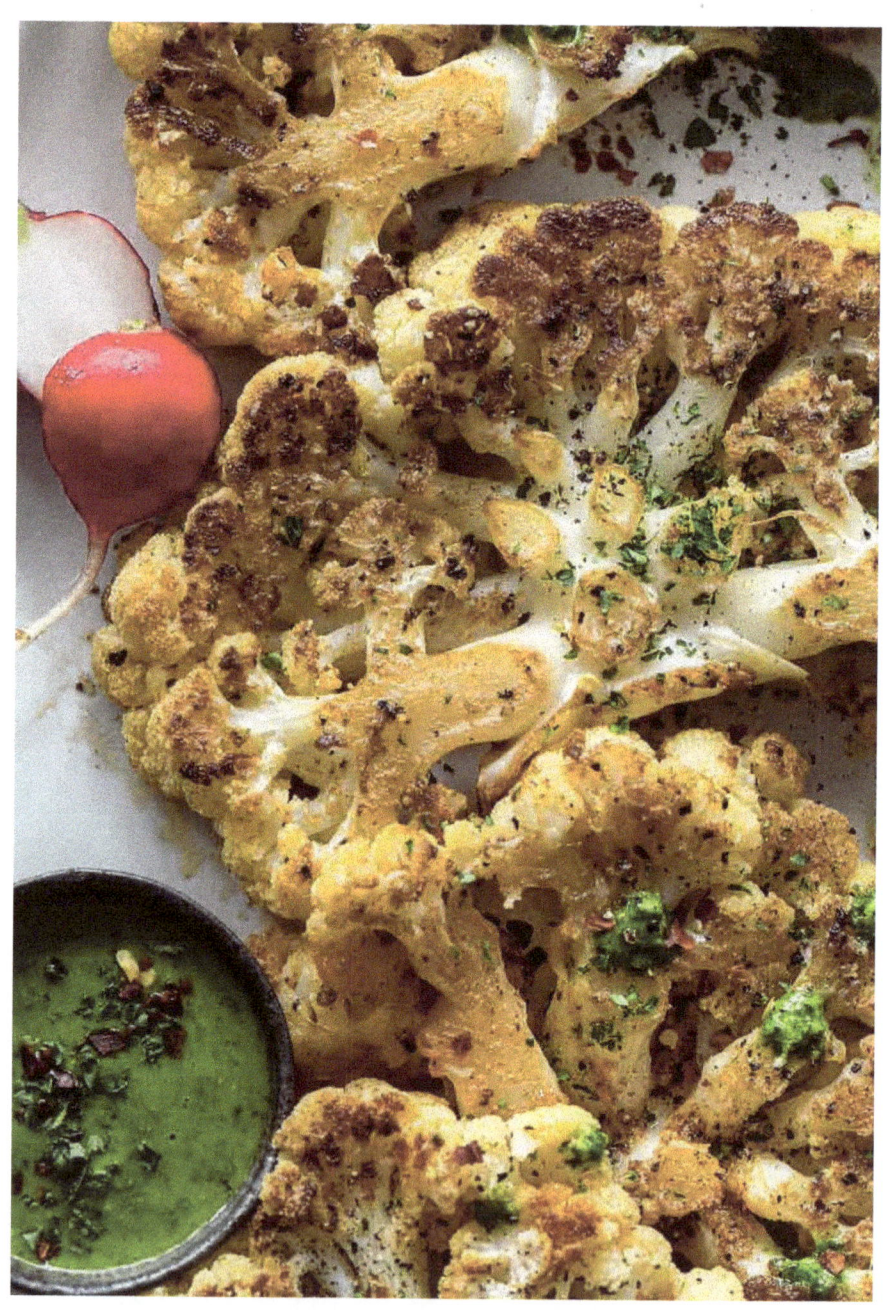

Cheddar, Squash 'n Zucchini Casserole

Servings per Recipe: 4

Cooking Time: 30 Minutes

Ingredients:

- 1 egg
- 5 saltine crackers, or when needed, crushed
- 2 tablespoons bread crumbs /30G
- 1/2-pound yellow squash, sliced /225G
- 1/2-pound zucchini, sliced /225G
- 1/2 cup shredded Cheddar cheese /65G
- 1-1/2 teaspoons white sugar /7.25G
- 1/2 teaspoon salt /2.5G
- 1/4 onion, diced
- 1/4 cup biscuit baking mix /32.5G
- 1/4 cup butter /32.5G

Instructions

1) Grease a baking pan that fits into your air fryer lightly with cooking spray. Add onion, zucchini, and yellow squash. Cover pan with foil and cook for 15 minutes at 360° F or 183°C or until tender.
2) Add salt, sugar, egg, butter, baking mix, and cheddar cheese. Mix well. Fold in crushed crackers. Top with bread crumbs.

3) Cook for 15 minutes at 390° F or 199°C until tops are lightly browned.
4) Dish out and enjoy.

Nutrition Information:

- Calories per Serving: 285
- Carbs: 16.4g
- Protein: 8.6g
- Fat: 20.5g

Cheesy BBQ Tater Tot

Servings per Recipe: 6

Cooking Time: 20 minutes

Ingredients:

- ½ cup shredded Cheddar /65G
- 12 slices of bacon
- 1-lb frozen tater tots, defrosted /450G
- 2 tbsp. chives /30G
- Ranch dressing, for serving

Instructions:

1) Thread one end of the strip of bacon on a steel skewer, thread a tater tot, and then flip the bacon over the tater tot, pushing it down the skewer. Repeat until you have a twirling bacon-and-tot.
2) Place skewer in your air fryer and cook for 10 minutes at 360° F or 183°C. Turn over skewer regularly while cooking.
3) Serve skewers on a plate, sprinkle cheese and chives on it.
4) Use ranch dressing for the side.

Nutrition Information:

- Calories per Serving: 337
- Carbs: 17.2g

- Protein: 11.5g
- Fat: 29.1g

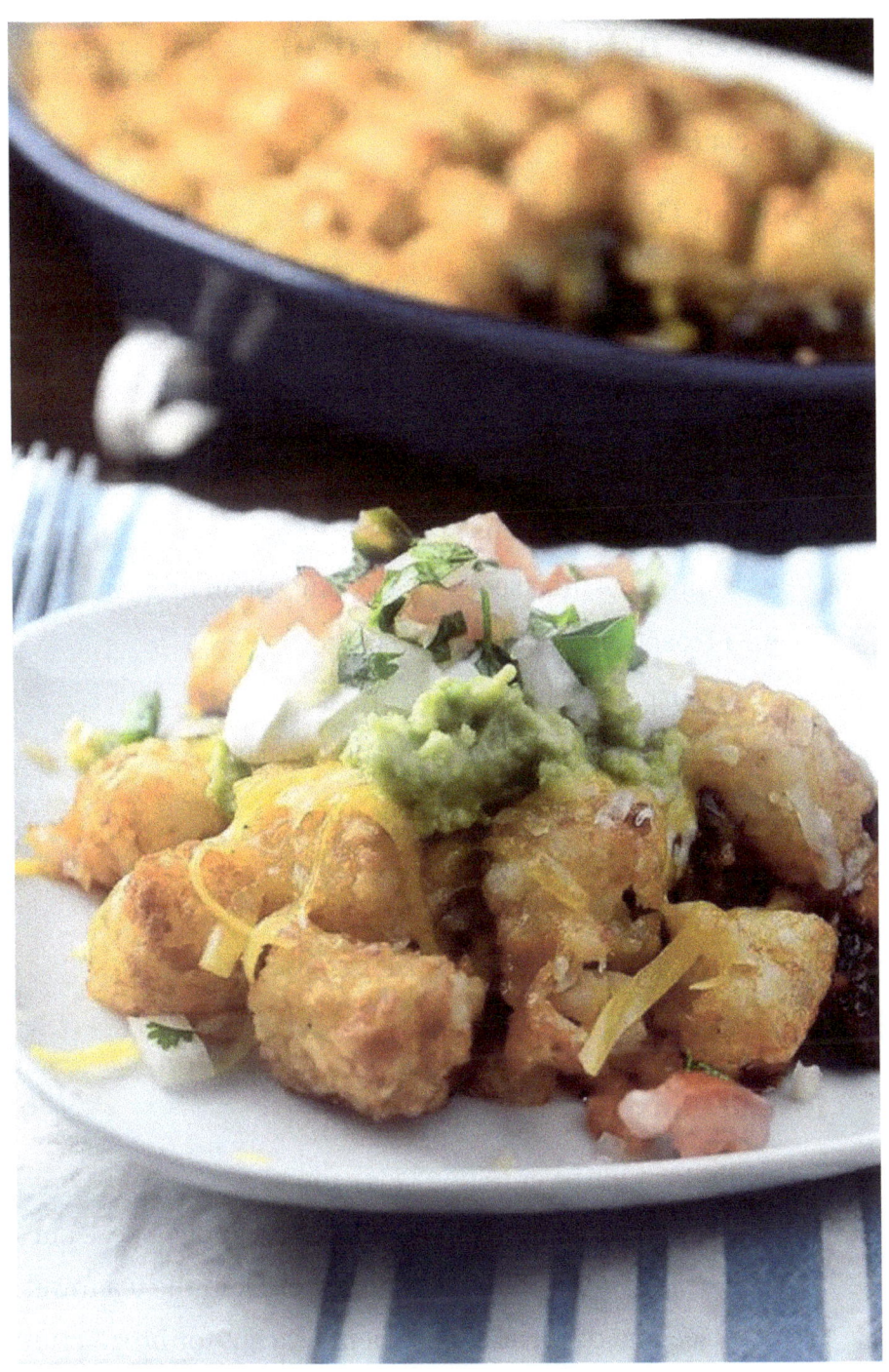

Chives 'n Thyme Spiced Veggie Burger

Serves: 8

Cooking Time: 15

Ingredients:

- ¼ cup desiccated coconut /32.5G
- ½ cup oats /65G
- ½ pound cauliflower, steamed and diced /225G
- 1 cup bread crumbs /130G
- 1 flax egg (1 flaxseed egg + 3 tablespoon or 45ML water)
- 1 teaspoon mustard powder /5G
- 2 teaspoons chives /10G
- 2 teaspoons coconut oil melted /10ML
- 2 teaspoons garlic, minced /10G
- 2 teaspoons parsley /10G
- 2 teaspoons thyme /10G
- 3 tablespoons plain flour/45G
- salt and pepper to taste

Instructions:

1) Preheat air fryer to 390° F or 199°C .
2) Place cauliflower in a large tea towel and squeeze out surplus water. Remove cauliflower from the tea towel and place in a bowl, add ingredients except for bread crumbs. Mix well.

3) Using your hands make 8 burger patties.
4) Turn the patties in bread crumbs, place them in the air fryer basket and avoid overlapping.
5) Cook until patties are crisp.

Nutrition information:

- Calories per serving: 70
- Carbohydrates: 10.85g
- Protein: 2.51g
- Fat: 1.85g

Coconut Battered Cauliflower Bites

Serves: 4

Cooking Time: 20 Minutes

Ingredients:

- salt and pepper to taste
- 1 flax egg (1 tablespoon flaxseed meal or 15G + 3 tablespoon or 45ML water)
- 1 small cauliflower, cut into florets
- 1 teaspoon mixed spice /5G
- ½ teaspoon mustard powder /2.5G
- 2 tablespoons maple syrup /30ML
- 1 clove of garlic, minced
- 2 tablespoons soy sauce /30ML
- 1/3 cup oats flour /43G
- 1/3 cup plain flour /43G
- 1/3 cup desiccated coconut /43G

Instructions

1) Preheat mid-air fryer to 400° F or 205°C.
2) Add oats, flour, and desiccated coconut in a bowl and mix well. Season with salt and pepper and allow to set.
3) Place flax egg in a bowl, add a pinch of salt and set aside.
4) Place cauliflower (florets) in a bowl, add mixed spice and mustard powder. Mix well.

5) Drench the florets inside the flax egg and then turn them over in the flour mixture.
6) Place inside air fryer basket and cook for 15 minutes.
7) Place a large saucepan over medium heat, add maple syrup, garlic, and soy sauce. Allow to boil until the sauce thickens.
8) Remove the florets from the air fryer pour them inside the saucepan. Turn the florets to coat, place in mid-air fryer and cook again for 5 more minutes.

Nutrition information:

- Calories per serving: 154
- Carbohydrates: 27.88g
- Protein: 4.69g
- Fat:2.68 g

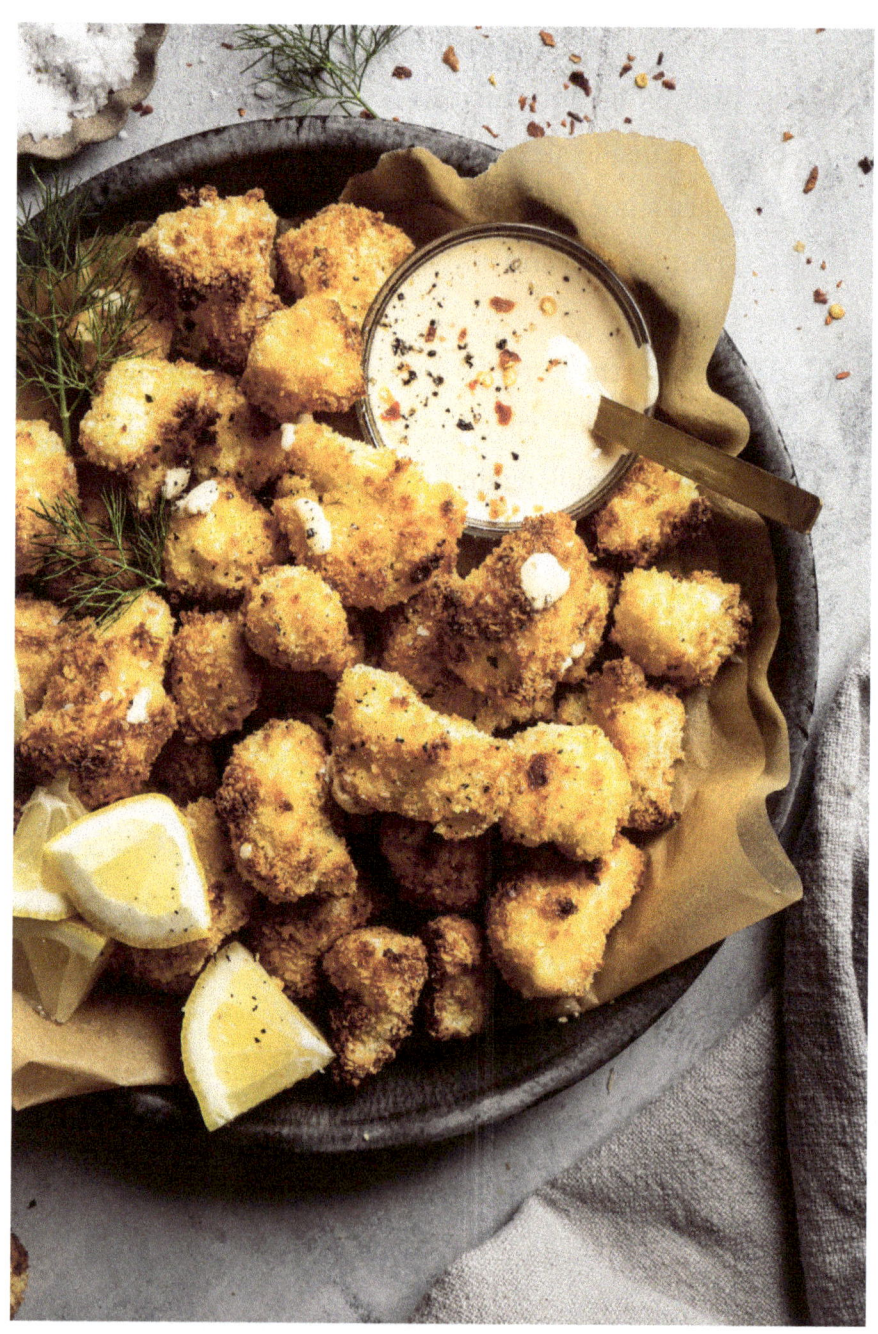

Creamy 'n Cheese Broccoli Bake

Servings per Recipe: 2

Cooking Time: 30 Minutes

Ingredients:

- 1-pound fresh broccoli, coarsely chopped /450G
- 2 tablespoons all-purpose flour /43G
- salt to taste
- 1 tablespoon dry bread crumbs /15G
- 1/2 large onion, coarsely chopped
- 1/2 (14 ounces or 120G) can evaporated milk, divided
- 1/2 cup cubed sharp Cheddar cheese /65G
- 1-1/2 teaspoons butter /7.5G
- 1/4 cup water /62.5ML

Instructions:

1) Oil baking pan lightly with cooking spray. Add milk and flour to the pan and cook for 5 minutes at 360° F or 183°C. After cooking add broccoli and the remaining milk. Mix well and cook for another 5 minutes.
2) Add in cheese and mix well until melted.
3) Add butter and bread crumbs to a small bowl. Sprinkle these on top of broccoli.
4) Cook for 20 Minutes at 360° F or 183°C or until tops are lightly browned.

5) Dish out and enjoy.

Nutrition Information:

- Calories per Serving: 444
- Carbs: 37.3g
- Protein: 23.1g
- Fat: 22.4g

Creole Seasoned Vegetables

Servings per Recipe: 5

Cooking Time: 15 minutes

Ingredients:

- ¼ cup honey /62.5ML
- ¼ cup yellow mustard /32.5G
- 1 large red bell pepper, sliced
- 1 teaspoon black pepper /5G
- 1 teaspoon salt /5G
- 2 large yellow squash, cut into ½ inch thick slices
- 2 medium zucchinis, cut into ½ inch thick slices
- 2 teaspoons creole seasoning /10G
- 2 teaspoons smoked paprika /10G
- 3 tablespoons olive oil /45ML

Instructions:

1) Preheat mid-air fryer to 330° F or 166°C.
2) Set the grill pan in the mid-air fryer.
3) Grab a Ziploc bag, add zucchini, squash, red bell pepper, extra virgin olive oil, salt and pepper. Shake the bag vigorously so that all vegetables are seasoned.
4) Place on the grill pan and cook for 15 minutes.

5) For the sauce, add mustard, honey, paprika, and creole seasoning. Mix well. Season with salt to taste.
6) Dish out the vegetables and dress using the sauce.

Nutrition information:

- Calories per serving: 164
- Carbs: 21.5g
- Protein: 2.6g
- Fat: 8.9g

Crisped Baked Cheese Stuffed Chile Pepper

Servings per Recipe: 3

Cooking Time: 30 Minutes

Ingredients:

- 1 (7 ounces or 210G) can whole green Chile peppers, drained
- 1 egg, beaten
- 1 tablespoon all-purpose flour /15G
- 1/2 (5 ounces or 150ML) can evaporated milk
- 1/2 (large) can tomato sauce
- 1/4-pound Monterey Jack cheese, shredded /112.5G
- 1/4-pound Longhorn or Cheddar cheese, shredded /112.5G
- 1/4 cup milk /62.5ML

Instructions:

1) Grease baking pan, evenly spread chilies on the pan, sprinkle cheddar and Jack cheese on the top.
2) Whisk flour, milk, and eggs in a bowl and pour over chilies.
3) Cook for 20 minutes at 360° F or 183°C.
4) Add tomato sauce on top.

5) Cook for 10 minutes at 390° F or 199°C or until the tops are lightly brown.
6) Dish out and enjoy.

Nutrition Information:

- Calories per Serving: 392
- Carbs: 12.0g
- Protein: 23.9g
- Fat: 27.6g

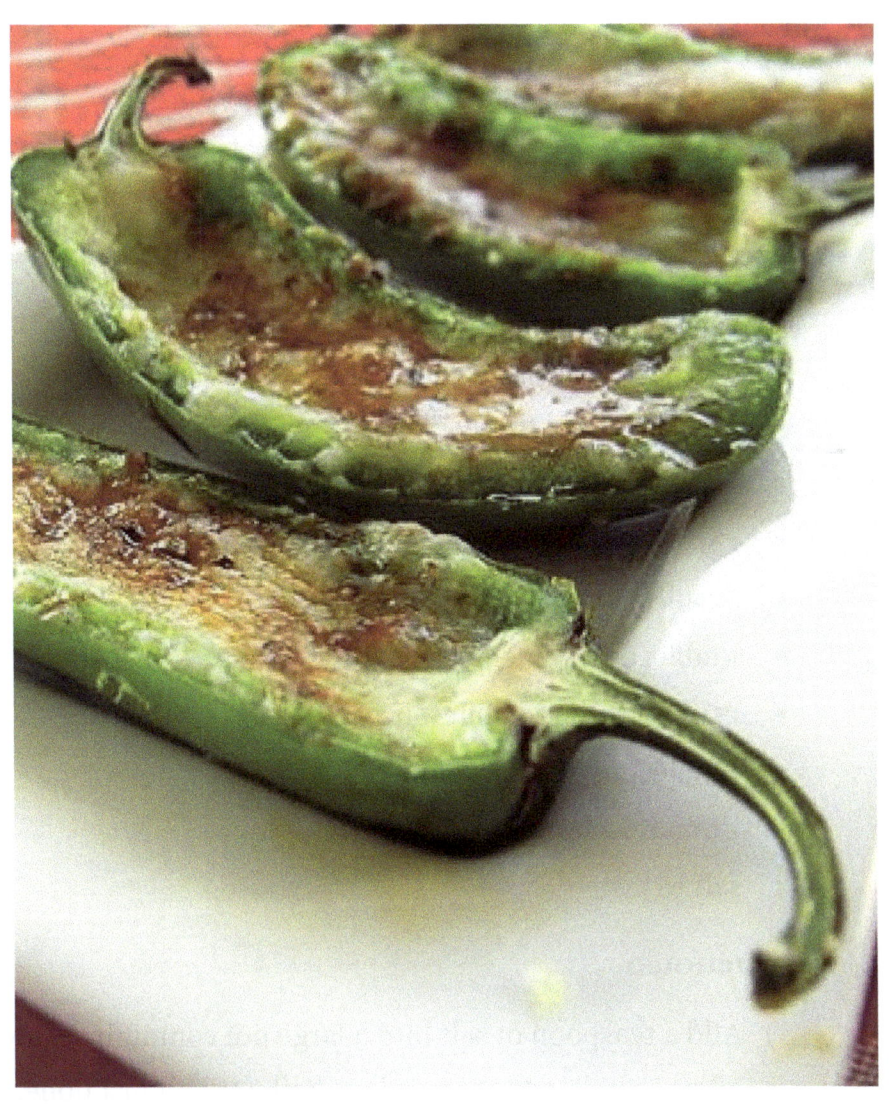

Crisped Noodle Salad Chinese Style

Serves: 2

Cooking Time: 20 minutes

Ingredients:

- 1 carrot, sliced thinly
- 1 cup cabbage, sliced thinly /130G
- 1 green bell pepper, sliced thinly
- 1 onion, sliced thinly
- 1 package wheat noodles
- 1 sprig coriander, chopped
- 1 tablespoon olive oil /15ML
- 1 tablespoon lime juice /15ML
- 1 tablespoon red chili sauce /15ML
- 1 tablespoon tamari /15G
- 1 tomato, chopped
- salt to taste

Instructions:

1) Add a teaspoon of salt into a large pot containing water, allow to boil, add the noodles, boil until almost done. Drain with a sieve.
2) Coat noodles evenly with oil.
3) lay the air fryer basket with a thin foil and put the coated noodles inside.

4) Meanwhile, preheat the air fryer to 395° F or 202°C. Place the basket in the air fryer for 15 to 20 minutes or cook until crisp. Place in a bowl.
5) In the meantime, add the tamari, red chili sauce, and lime juice to a bowl and mix well. Season with salt and pepper to taste.
6) Add the vegetables and pour sauce over the mid air-fried noodles.

Nutrition information:

- Calories per serving: 165
- Carbohydrates: 20.41g
- Protein:4.12 g
- Fat:7.39 g

Crisped Tofu with Paprika

Serves: 4

Ingredients:

- ¼ cup cornstarch /32.5G
- 1 block extra firm tofu, pressed to remove excess water and cut into cubes
- 1 tablespoon smoked paprika /15G
- salt and pepper to taste

Instructions:

1) Line air fryer basket with aluminium foil and brush with oil.
2) Preheat air fryer to 370° F or 188°C.
3) Mix all ingredients in the bowl. Toss to blend.
4) Place in the air fryer basket and cook for 12 minutes.

Nutrition information:

- Calories per serving: 155
- Carbohydrates: 11.56 g
- Protein: 11.74 g
- Fat: 6.88 g

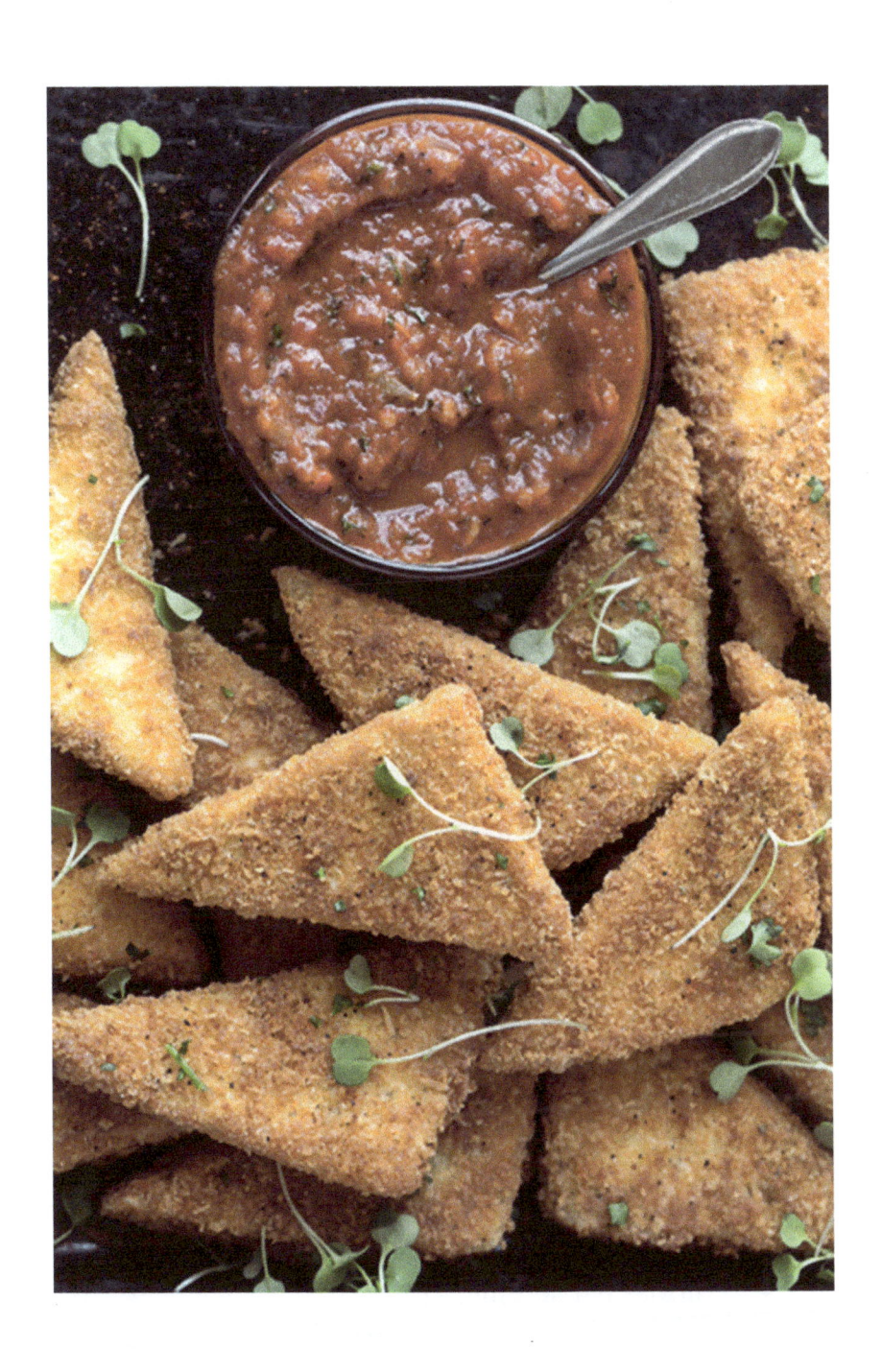

Crispy 'n Healthy Avocado Fingers

Serves: 4

Cooking Time: 10 Minutes

Ingredients:

- ½ cup panko breadcrumbs /65G
- ½ teaspoon salt /2.5G
- 1 pitted Haas avocado, peeled and sliced
- liquid from 1 can of white beans or aquafaba

Instructions:

1) Preheat mid-air fryer at 350° F or 177°C.
2) Mix the breadcrumbs and salt in a bowl until well combined.
3) Dip the avocado slices inside the aquafaba and then in the breadcrumb mixture.
4) Place the avocado slices one after the other in a single layer in the air fryer basket.
5) Cook for 10 minutes and shake frequently for even doneness.

Nutrition information:

- Calories per serving: 51
- Carbohydrates: 6.45g
- Protein: 1.39g

- Fat: 7.51g

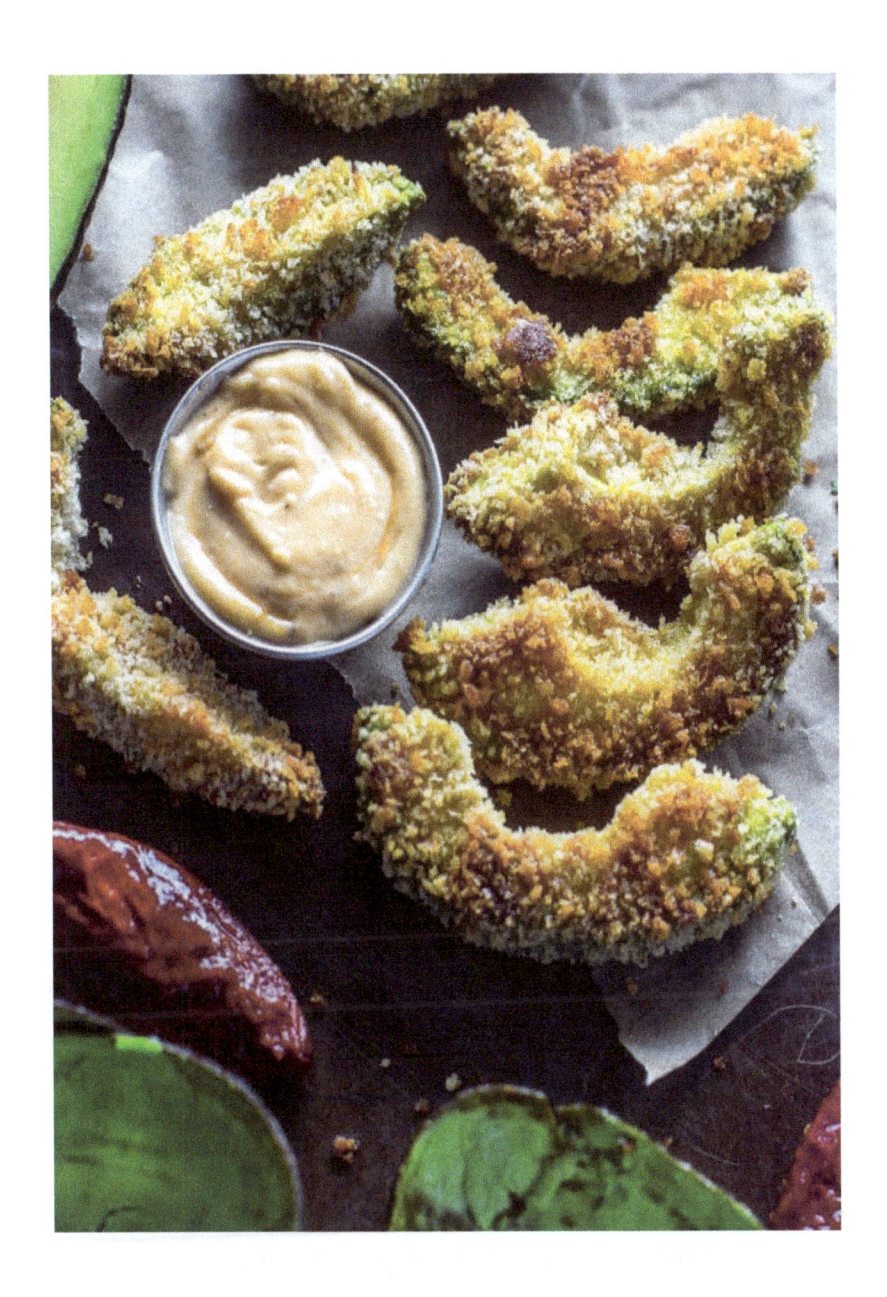

Crispy 'n Savory Spring Rolls

Serves: 4

Cooking Time: 15

Ingredients:

- ½ teaspoon ginger, finely chopped /2.5G
- 1 celery stalk, chopped
- 1 cup shiitake mushroom, sliced thinly /65G
- 1 medium carrot, shredded
- 1 tablespoon soy sauce /15ML
- 1 teaspoon coconut sugar /5G
- 1 teaspoon corn starch + 2 tablespoon water /5G + 30ML
- 1 teaspoon nutritional yeast /5G
- 8 spring roll wrappers

Instructions:

1) Mix the celery stalk, carrots, ginger, coconut sugar, soy sauce and nutritional yeast properly.
2) Place a tablespoon of vegetable oil in the middle of the spring roll wrappers.
3) Roll and seal the edges of the wrapper using the cornstarch mixture.
4) Cook in a preheated air fryer to 400° F or 205°C for 15 or until the spring roll wrapper is crispy.

Nutrition information:

- Calories per serving: 118
- Carbohydrates: 15g
- Protein: 10g
- Fat: 2g

Crispy Asparagus Dipped in Paprika-Garlic Spice

Serves: 5

Cooking Time: 15 minutes

Ingredients:

- ¼ cup almond flour /32.5G
- ½ teaspoon garlic powder /2.5G
- ½ teaspoon smoked paprika /2.5G
- 10 medium asparagus, trimmed
- 2 large eggs, beaten
- 2 tablespoons parsley, chopped /30G
- Salt and pepper to taste

Instructions:

1) Preheat the air fryer for 5 minutes.
2) Add the parsley, garlic powder, almond flour, and smoked paprika to a bowl and mix properly. Season with salt and pepper.
3) Dip the asparagus in the whisked eggs and turnover in the almond flour mixture to coat evenly.
4) Place in air fryer basket.
5) Cook for 15 at 350° F or 177°C.

Nutrition information:

- Calories per serving: 114
- Carbohydrates: 4.9g
- Protein: 5.2g
- Fat: 8.2g

Crispy Fry Green Tomatoes

Servings per Recipe: 1

Cooking Time: 7 minutes

Ingredients:

- ½ cup panko bread crumbs /65G
- ½ teaspoon cooking oil /2.5ML
- ½ teaspoon dried basil, ground /2.5G
- ½ teaspoon dried oregano, ground /2.5G
- ½ teaspoon granulated onion /2.5G
- 1 medium-sized green tomato, sliced
- 3 tablespoons cornstarch /45G
- Salt and pepper to taste

Instructions:

1) Combine the panko bread crumbs, cornstarch, basil, oregano, onion, salt and pepper in na mixing bowl. Mix properly.
2) Dip the tomato slices in the bread crumb mixture.
3) Sprinkle with oil and place the dredged tomatoes in the double layer rack.
4) Place in the air fryer.
5) Cook for 7 minutes at 330° F or 166°C.

Nutrition information:

- Calories per serving: 260
- Carbs: 54.1g
- Protein: 5.4g
- Fat: 3.4g

Crispy Onion Seasoned with Paprika 'n Cajun

Serves: 4

Cooking Time: 20 Minutes

Ingredients:

- ¼ cup coconut milk /62.5ML
- ½ teaspoon Cajun seasoning /2.5G
- ¾ cup almond flour /88G
- 1 ½ teaspoon paprika /7.5G
- 1 large white onion
- 1 teaspoon garlic powder /5G
- 2 large eggs, beaten
- Salt and pepper to taste

Instructions:

1) Peel the onion
2) Add the coconut milk and the eggs to a mixing bowl and whisk well.
3) Soak the onion inside the egg mixture.
4) In another bowl, combine the almond flour, paprika garlic powder, Cajun seasoning, salt and pepper.
5) Dredge the onion in the almond flour mixture.
6) Grease with cooking spray.
7) Place in mid-air fryer.

8) Cook for 20 Minutes at 350° F or 177°C .

Nutrition information:

- Calories per serving: 93
- Carbohydrates: 6.7g
- Protein: 2.6g
- Fat: 6.2g

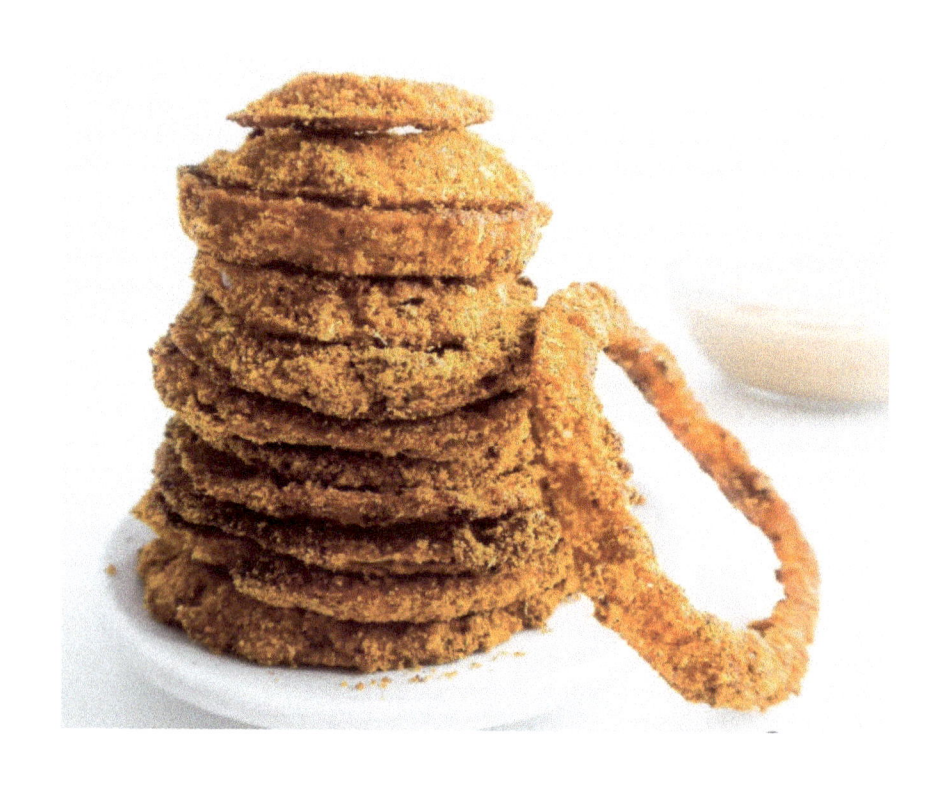

Crispy Vegetarian Ravioli

Serves: 4

Cooking Time: 6 minutes

Ingredients:

- ¼ cup aquafaba /62.5ML
- ½ cup panko bread crumbs /65G
- 1 teaspoon dried basil /5G
- 1 teaspoon dried oregano /5G
- 1 teaspoon garlic powder /5G
- 2 teaspoons nutritional yeast /10G
- 8-ounces vegan ravioli /240G
- cooking spray
- salt and pepper to taste

Instructions:

1) Lay aluminium foil within the air fryer basket and spray with oil.
2) Preheat the air fryer to 400° F or 205°C.
3) Add the panko bread crumbs, nutritional yeast, basil, oregano, and garlic powder to a bowl and mix properly. Season with salt and pepper to taste.
4) Squeeze the aquafaba in a bowl
5) Lightly cover the ravioli with the aquafaba and then turn over in the panko mixture.

6) Spray with oil and place in the air fryer.
7) Cook for 6 minutes ensuring you shake the mid-air fryer basket halfway through cooking time.

Nutrition information:

- Calories per serving: 82
- Carbohydrates: 12.18g
- Protein:3.36 g
- Fat: 2.15g

Crispy Veggie Tempura Style

Servings per Recipe: 3

Cooking Time: 15 minutes

Ingredients:

- ¼ teaspoon salt /1.25G
- ¾ cup club soda /188ML
- 1 ½ cups panko bread crumbs /195G
- 1 cup broccoli florets /130G
- 1 egg, beaten
- 1 red bell pepper, cut into strips
- 1 small sweet potato, peeled and cut into thick slices
- 1 small zucchini, cut into thick slices
- 1/3 cup all-purpose flour /43G
- 2/3 cup cornstarch /87G
- Non-stick cooking spray

Instructions:

1) Lightly cover the vegetables with cornstarch and also in the all-purpose flour mixture.
2) Dip each vegetable in the blend of egg and club soda before dredging in bread crumbs.
3) Place the vegetables on the double layer rack and brush with cooking oil.
4) Place inside the air fryer.

5) Close and cook for 20 minutes at 330° F or 166°C .

Nutrition information:

- Calories per serving:277
- Carbs: 51.6g
- Protein: 7.2g
- Fat: 4.2g

Crispy Wings with Lemony Old Bay Spice

Serves: 4

Cooking Time: 25 minutes

Ingredients:

- ½ cup butter /65G
- ¾ cup almond flour /88G
- 1 tablespoon old bay spices /15G
- 1 teaspoon lemon juice, freshly squeezed /5ML
- 3 pounds chicken wings /1350G
- Salt and pepper to taste

Instructions:

1) Warm up the air fryer for 5 minutes.
2) Combine all ingredients apart from the butter
3) Place in the air fryer basket.
4) Cook for 25 minutes at 350° F or 177°C .
5) Always shake the air fryer basket halfway through cooking.
6) Once cooked, drizzle with melted butter.

Nutrition information:

- Calories per serving: 750
- Carbohydrates: 1.6g
- Protein: 52.5g

- Fat: 59.2g

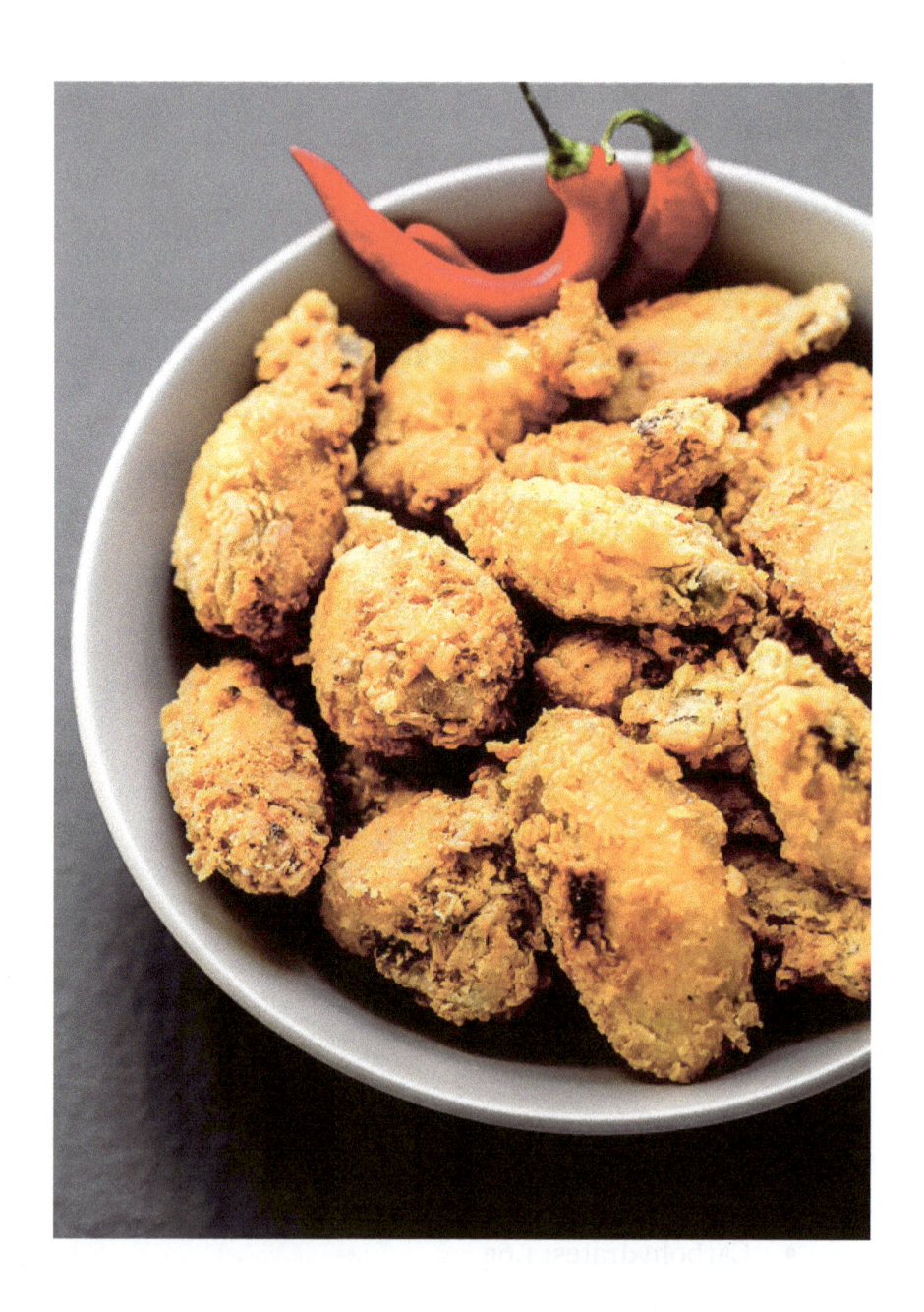

Curry 'n Coriander Spiced Bread Rolls

Serves: 5

Cooking Time: 15 minutes

Ingredients:

- ½ teaspoon mustard seeds /2.5G
- ½ teaspoon turmeric /2.5G
- 1 bunch coriander, chopped
- 1 tablespoon extra virgin olive oil /15ML
- 2 green chilies, seeded and chopped
- 2 small onions, chopped
- 2 sprigs, curry leaves
- 5 large potatoes, boiled
- 8 slices of vegan wheat bread, brown sides discarded
- salt and pepper to taste

Instructions:

1) Mash the potatoes in a bowl and season with salt and pepper. Set aside.

2) Over medium to low heat, heat extra virgin olive oil in a pan and add the mustard seeds. Stir before the seeds spit. Then add the onions and fry until translucent. Add the turmeric powder and curry leaves, and then stir. Continue to cook for just two more minutes until the aroma saturates. Remove from heat and add the potatoes. Stir the content inside the green chilies and coriander.
3) Wet the bread and remove the excess water.
4) Place a tablespoon of the potato mixture in the middle of the bread and gently roll the bread in so the potato filling is entirely sealed in the bread.
5) Brush with oil, place in the mid-air fryer.
6) Cook for 15 mintues at 400° F or 205°C. Make sure to shake the mid-air fryer basket gently halfway from the cooking time.

Nutrition information:

- Calories per serving: 462
- Carbohydrates: 96.65g
- Protein: 11.3g
- Fat: 3.88g

Easy Baked Root Veggies

Serves: 4

Cooking Time: 45 minutes

Ingredients:

- ¼ cup organic olive oil /62.5ML
- 1 head broccoli, cut into florets
- 1 tablespoon dry onion powder /15G
- 2 sweet potatoes, peeled and cubed
- 4 carrots, cut into chunks
- 4 zucchinis, sliced thickly
- salt and pepper to taste

Instructions:

1) Preheat the air fryer to 400° F or 205°C .
2) Add all ingredients to a baking dish, mix properly. Bake for 45 minutes or before the vegetables are tender or when the sides have browned.

Nutrition information:

- Calories per serving: 310
- Carbohydrates: 41.05g
- Protein: 5.22g
- Fat: 13.93g

Easy Fry Portobello Mushroom

Servings per Recipe: 2

Cooking Time: 10

Ingredients:

- 1 tablespoon cooking oil /15ML
- 1-pound Portobello mushroom, sliced /450G
- Salt and pepper to taste

Instructions:

1) Place the grill pan in the air fryer.
2) Place all ingredients in a bowl and mix to coat. Add mushrooms and coat well.
3) Arrange the mushrooms in the grill pan. Place in the air fryer.
4) Cook for 10 minutes at 330° F or 166°C.

Nutrition information:

- Calories per serving: 135
- Carbs: 12.2g
- Protein: 7.8g
- Fat: 8.5g

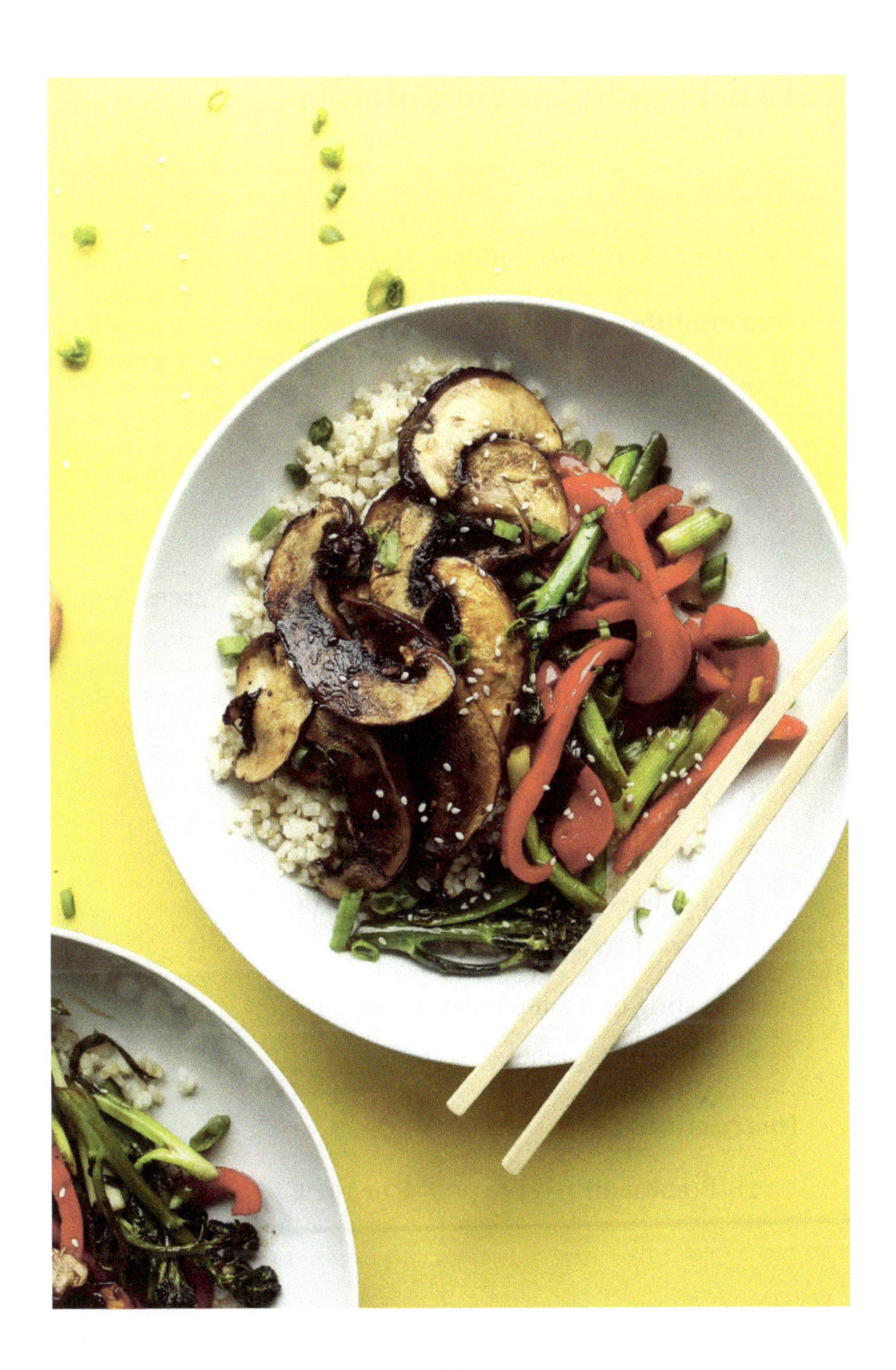

Egg-Less Spinach Quiche

Serves: 4

Cooking Time: 30 Minutes

Ingredients

- ½ cup cold coconut oil /125ML
- ½ tablespoon dried dill /2.5G
- ¾ cup wholemeal flour /88G
- 1 onion, chopped
- 1 package firm tofu, pressed to eliminate excess water then crumbled
- 1-pound spinach washed and chopped /450G
- 2 tablespoons cold water /30ML
- 2 tablespoons nutritional yeast /30G
- 2 tablespoons extra virgin olive oil /30ML
- 4 ounces mushrooms, sliced /120G
- a pinch of salt
- a sprig of fresh parsley, chopped
- salt and pepper

Instructions:

1) Preheat air fryer to 375° F or 191°C.

2) Sift the flour and salt together. Add the coconut oil before the flour dissolves. Add water gradually while kneading the dough until it forms a hard dough. Wrap the dough in cling film and place in the fridge to set for 30 minutes.
3) Heat extra virgin olive oil in a pan over medium heat and sauté the onion for 1 minute. Add the mushroom and tofu. Add the spinach, dried dill, and nutritional yeast. Season with salt and pepper to taste and lastly add the parsley. Set aside.
4) Roll the dough on a floured flat surface and form a thin dough. Place the dough in the greased baking pan. Pour the tofu mixture and cook for 30 minutes or until the pastry is crispy.

Nutrition information:

- Calories per serving: 531
- Carbohydrates: 49.37g
- Protein: 11.4g
- Fat: 35.22g

Fried Broccoli Recipe From India

Serves: 6

Cooking Time: 15

Ingredients

- ¼ teaspoon turmeric powder /1.25G
- ½ pounds broccoli, cut into florets /2.5G
- 1 tablespoon almond flour /15G
- 1 teaspoon garam masala /5G
- 2 tablespoons coconut milk /30ML
- ·Salt and pepper to taste

Instructions:

1) Preheat the air fryer for 5 minutes.
2) Mix all ingredients in a bowl. Coat the broccoli florets with the other ingredients.
3) Place the broccoli florets in an air fryer basket and cook for 15 minutes until crispy.

Nutrition information:

- Calories per serving: 96
- Carbohydrates: 8.9g
- Protein: 3.1g
- Fat: 6.9g

Fried Chickpea-Fig on Arugula

Serves: 4

Cooking Time: 20 minutes

Ingredients

- 1 ½ cups chickpeas, cooked /195G
- 1 teaspoon cumin seeds, roasted then crushed /5G
- 2 tablespoons extra-virgin essential olive oil /30ML
- 3 cups arugula rocket, washed and dried /390G
- 4 tablespoons balsamic vinegar /60ML
- 8 fresh figs, halved
- salt and pepper to taste

Instructions

1) Preheat air fryer to 375° F or 191°C.
2) Line the air fryer basket with aluminium foil and brush with oil.
3) Place the figs inside the air fryer and cook for 10 minutes.
4) Mix the chickpeas and cumin seeds in a bowl properly.
5) Cook the chickpeas for 10 minutes. Allow to cool
6) Combine the balsamic vinegar, organic olive oil, salt and pepper in a bowl and mix well.
7) Place the arugula rocket in a salad bowl and add the cooled figs and chickpeas.

8) Pour the sauce over the content of the salad bowl and mix to coat.
9) Serve immediately.

Nutrition information:

- Calories per serving: 388
- Carbohydrates: 62.51g
- Protein:16.72 g
- Fat:7.92 g

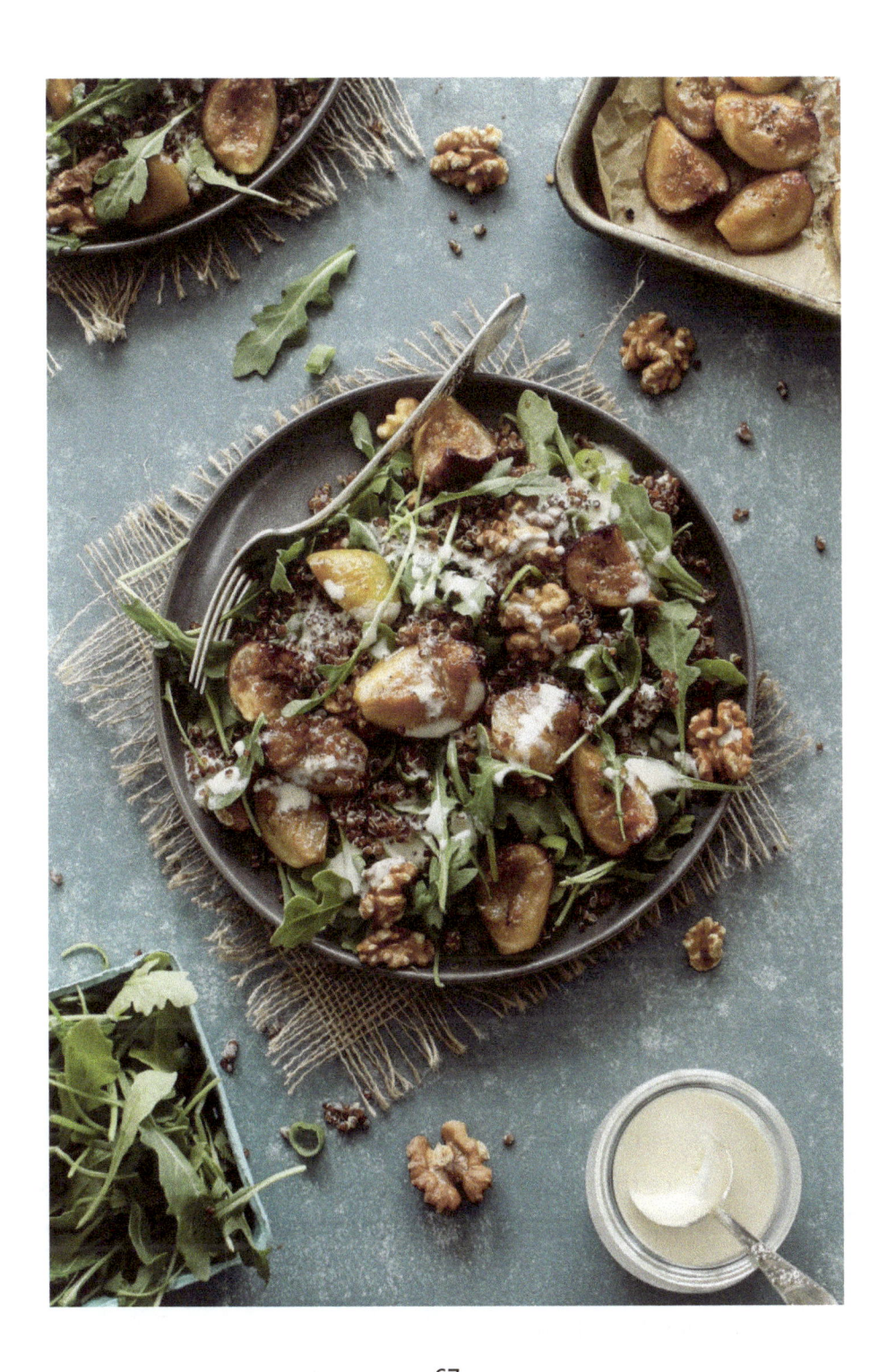

Fried Falafel Recipe from the Middle East

Serves: 8

Cooking Time: 15

Ingredients:

- ¼ cup coriander, chopped /32.5G
- ¼ cup parsley, chopped /32.5G
- ½ onion, diced
- ½ teaspoon coriander seeds /2.5G
- ½ teaspoon red pepper flakes /2.5G
- ½ teaspoon salt /2.5G
- 1 tablespoon juice from freshly squeezed lemon /15ML
- 1 teaspoon cumin seeds /5G
- 2 cups chickpeas from can, drained and rinsed /260G
- ·3 cloves garlic
- 3 tablespoons all-purpose flour /45G
- cooking spray

Instructions:

1) Place a pan over a medium heat, toast the cumin and coriander seeds until scented.
2) Place the toasted seeds in a mortar and crush the seeds.
3) Place all ingredients aside from the cooking spray in a blender. Add the toasted cumin and coriander seeds.
4) Blend until fine.

5) Shape the amalgamation into falafels and spray olive oil.
6) Place within a preheated air fryer and make sure that they don't overlap.
7) Cook at 400° F or 205°C for 15 minutes or until the surface becomes golden brown.

Nutrition information:

- Calories per serving: 110
- Carbohydrates: 18.48g
- Protein: 5.11g
- Fat: 1.72g

Fried Tofu Recipe from Malaysia

Servings per Recipe: 4

Cooking Time: 30 Minutes

Ingredients:

- 1 block tofu, cut into strips
- 1 tablespoon maple syrup /15ML
- 1 teaspoon sriracha sauce /5ML
- 2 cloves of garlic
- 2 tablespoons soy sauce /30ML
- 2 teaspoons fresh ginger no need to peel, coarsely chopped /10G
- juice of just one fresh lime

- Peanut Butter Sauce Ingredients

- 1 tablespoon soy sauce /15ML
- 1/2 cup creamy peanut butter /65G
- 1-2 teaspoons Sriracha sauce to taste /10ML
- 2 cloves of garlic
- 2-inch little bit of fresh ginger coarsely chopped
- 6 tablespoons of water /90ML
- juice of merely one/2 a fresh lemon

Instructions:

1) Blend all peanut butter sauce ingredients until smooth and creamy. Transfer into a medium bowl and place aside for dipping sauce.
2) Blend garlic, sriracha, ginger, maple syrup, lime juice, and soy sauce until smooth. Pour into a bowl and add strips of tofu, Marinate for 30 minutes.
3) Skewer tofu strips.
4) Place on skewer rack and air fry for 15 at 370° F or 188°C.
5) Serve and enjoy.

Nutrition Information:

- Calories per Serving: 347
- Carbs: 16.6g
- Protein: 16.6g
- Fat: 23.8g

Garlic 'n Basil Crackers

Serves: 6

Cooking Time: 15 minutes

Ingredients:

- ¼ teaspoon dried basil powder /1.25G
- ½ teaspoon baking powder /2.5G
- 1 ¼ cups almond flour /162.5G
- 1 clove of garlic, minced
- 3 tablespoons coconut oil /45ML
- A pinch of red pepper cayenne powder
- Salt and pepper to taste

Instructions:

1) Preheat the air fryer for 5 minutes.
2) Mix everything in a mixing bowl to make a dough.
3) Transfer the dough to a clean and flat surface and knead until 2mm thick. Cut into squares.
4) Place gently in mid-air fryer basket. Do this in batches if you like.
5) Cook for 15 minutes at 325° F or 163°C.

Nutrition information:

- Calories per serving: 206
- Carbohydrates: 2.9g

- Protein: 5.3g
- Fat: 19.3g

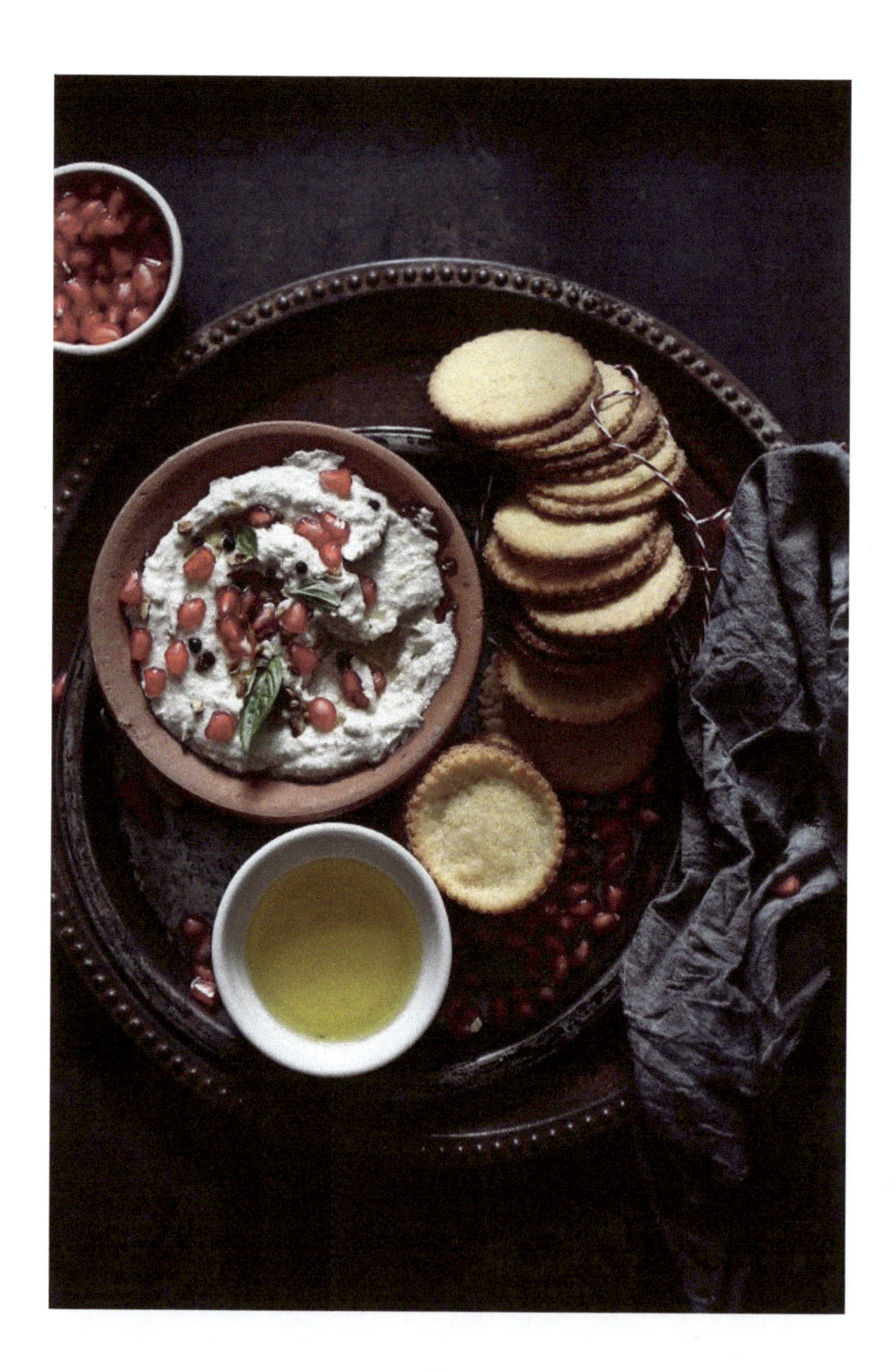

Garlic-Wine Flavored Vegetables

Servings per Recipe: 4

Cooking Time: 15 minutes

Ingredients:

- ¼ cup chopped fresh basil /32.5G
- 1 ½ tablespoons honey1 teaspoon Dijon mustard /22.5ML + 5G
- 1 cup baby portobello mushrooms, chopped
- 1 package frozen chopped vegetables
- 1 red onion, sliced
- 1/3 cup olive oil /188ML
- 3 tablespoons dark wine vinegar /45ML
- 4 cloves of garlic, minced
- Salt and pepper to taste

Instructions:

1) Preheat the air fryer to 330° F or 166°C.
2) Place the grill pan in the air fryer.
3) Add the vegetables and season with salt, pepper, and garlic in a Ziploc bag. Shake well to combine evenly.
4) Place on the grill pan and cook for 15 minutes.
5) Combine the remaining portion of the ingredients in a bowl and season with more salt and pepper.

6) Sprinkle the grilled vegetables using the sauce.

Nutrition information:

- Calories per serving: 200
- Carbs: 8.3g
- Protein: 2.1g
- Fat: 18.2g

Grilled 'n Glazed Strawberries

Servings per Recipe: 2

Cooking Time: 20 minutes

Ingredients:

- 1 tbsp honey /15ML
- 1 tsp lemon zest /5G
- 1-lb large strawberries /450G
- 3 tbsp melted butter /45ML
- Lemon wedges
- Pinch kosher salt

Instructions:

1) Thread the strawberries in 4 skewers.
2) Mix the remaining Ingredients aside from the lemon wedges well. Brush these mixed ingredients around the strawberries.
3) Place the skewers on the air fryer skewer rack.
4) For 10 Minutes, cook at 360° F or 183°C. Halfway through cooking time, brush with honey mixture and turnover skewer.
5) Serve and squeeze the lemon on the skewer to dress.

Nutrition Information:

- Calories per Serving: 281

- Carbs: 27.9g
- Protein: 1.8g
- Fat: 18.0g

Grilled 'n Spiced Tomatoes on Garden Salad

Servings per Recipe: 4

Cooking Time: 20 Minutes

Ingredients:

- ¼ cup golden raisings /32.5G
- ¼ cup hazelnuts, toasted and chopped /32.5G
- ¼ cup pistachios, toasted and chopped /32.5G
- ½ cup chopped chives /65G
- ¾ cup cilantro leaves, chopped /88G
- ¾ cup fresh parsley, chopped /88G
- 1 clove of garlic, minced
- 2 tablespoons white balsamic vinegar /30ML
- 3 large green tomatoes
- 4 leaves iceberg lettuce
- 5 tablespoons olive oil /75ML
- ·Salt and pepper to taste

Instructions

1) Preheat mid-air fryer to 330° F or 166°C.
2) Place the grill pan in the mid-air fryer.
3) Add the tomatoes with garlic, oil, salt and pepper to taste into a mixing bowl and mix well.

4) Place on the grill pan and grill for 20 minutes.
5) Remove from the air fryer, place in a salad bowl with the rest of the ingredients.

Nutrition information:

- Calories per serving: 287
- Carbs: 12.2g
- Protein: 4.8g
- Fat: 25.9g

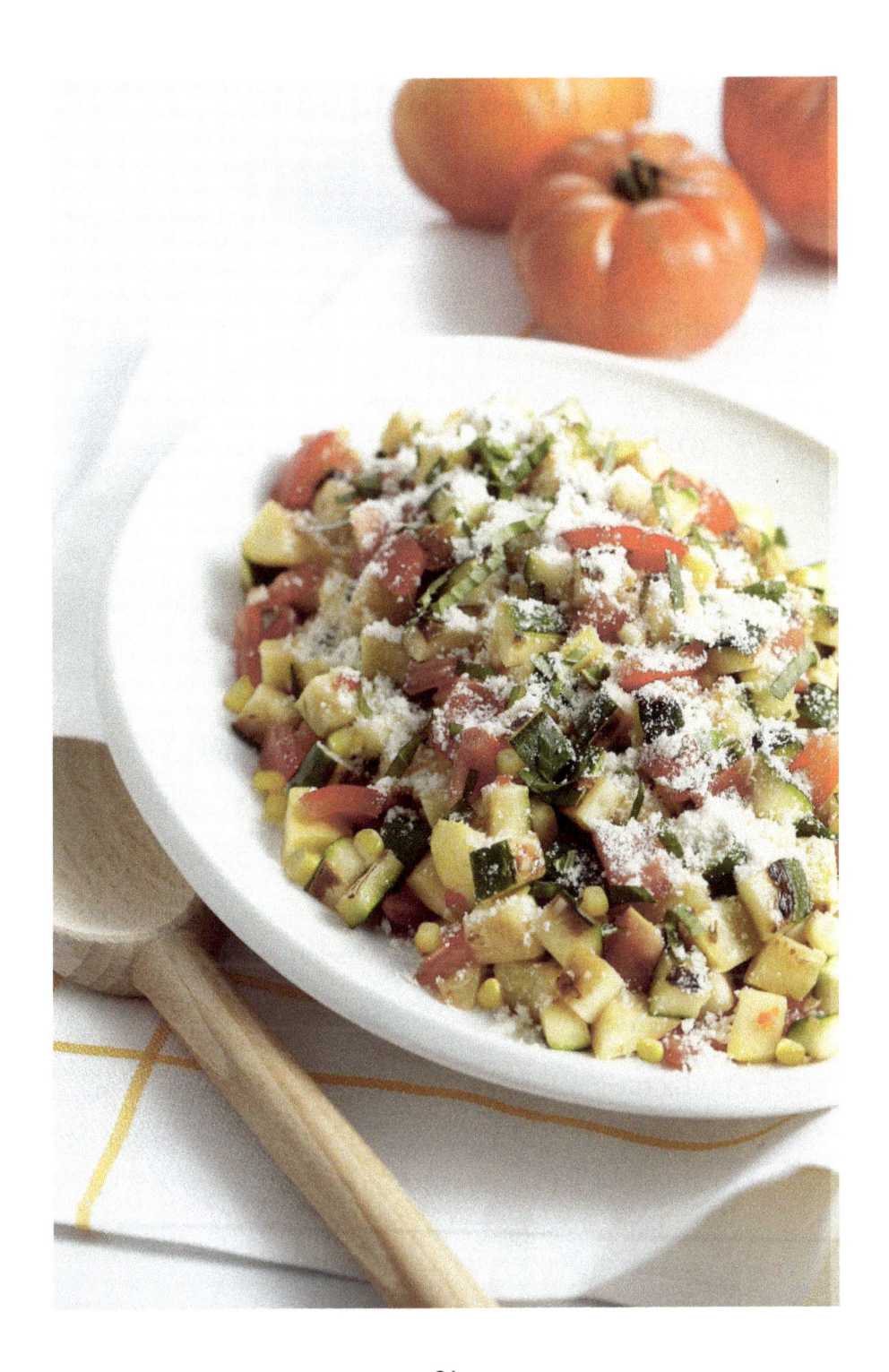

Grilled Drunken Mushrooms

Servings per Recipe: 4

Cooking Time: 20 Minutes

Ingredients:

- 2 garlic cloves, finely chopped
- 3 tablespoons chopped fresh thyme and/or rosemary leaves /45G
- Large pinch of crushed red pepper flakes
- 1 teaspoon kosher salt, and many more to taste /5G
- 6 scallions, cut crosswise into 2-inch pieces
- 1-pint cherry tomatoes /473G
- 1-pint cremini, button, or other small mushrooms /473G
- 1/2 cup extra-virgin essential olive oil /125ML
- ·1/2 teaspoon freshly ground black pepper, plus more to taste /2.5G
- 1/4 cup red wine or Sherry vinegar /62.5ML

Instructions:

1) Mix the black pepper, salt, red pepper flakes, thyme, vinegar, oil, and garlic in a Ziploc bag. Add mushrooms, tomatoes, and scallions. Mix well and allow it to marinate for half one hour.

2) Thread mushrooms, tomatoes, and scallions on a skewer. Reserve sauce for basting. Place on skewer rack in the air fryer. If needed, cook in batches.
3) For 10 Minutes, cook on 360° F or 183°C . Halfway through cooking time, turnover skewers and baste with reserved sauce.
4) Serve and enjoy.

Nutrition Information:

- Calories per Serving: 126
- Carbs: 4.1g
- Protein: 1.0g
- Fat: 11.7g

Grilled Eggplant with Cumin-Paprika Spice

Servings per Recipe: 2

Cooking Time: 20 minutes

Ingredients:

- 1 Chinese eggplant, sliced into 1-inch thick circles
- 1 medium bell pepper, cut into chunks
- 1 tablespoon coriander seeds /15G
- 1 tablespoon essential olive oil /15ML
- 1 teaspoon cumin /5G
- ·1 teaspoon paprika /5G
- 1 teaspoon salt /5G
- ·1 zucchini, sliced into 1-inch thick circles
- 3 garlic cloves

Instructions:

1) Blend garlic, coriander, olive oil, cumin, paprika, and salt until creamy.
2) Thread bell pepper, eggplant, and zucchini in skewers. Brush with the garlic creamy paste. Place on skewer rack in the air fryer.

3) For 10 Minutes, cook on 360**O** F or 183°C. Halfway through cooking time, turnover skewers. If needed, cook in batches.

4) Serve and enjoy.

Nutrition Information:

- Calories per Serving: 181
- Carbs: 22.4g
- Protein: 4.2g
- Fat: 8.2g

Grilled Olive-Tomato with Dill-Parsley Oil

Servings per Recipe: 6

Cooking Time: 16 minutes

Ingredients:

- 1 big block of feta (about 12-oz.), cut into cubes
- 1 tbsp lemon juice /15ML
- 1 clove garlic, smashed
- 1 tbsp Chopped fresh dill /15G
- 1 tbsp chopped fresh parsley /15G
- Flaky sea salt
- ·Freshly ground black pepper
- 12 pitted kalamata olives
- 12 cherry tomatoes
- 1 cucumber, cut into 12 large cubes
- 1/4 cup extra-virgin essential olive oil /62.5ML

Instructions:

1) Mix parsley, dill, garlic, lemon juice, and extra virgin olive oil in a bowl. Season with pepper and salt. Add feta cheese and allow to marinate for at least 15 minutes.

2) Thread feta, olives, cherry tomatoes, and cucumber in skewers. Place on skewer rack in the air fryer. If needed, cook in batches.
3) Cook for 8 minutes at 390° F or 199°C.
4) Serve and get.

Nutrition Information:

- Calories per Serving: 217
- Carbs: 7.1g
- Protein: 8.8g
- Fat: 17.0g

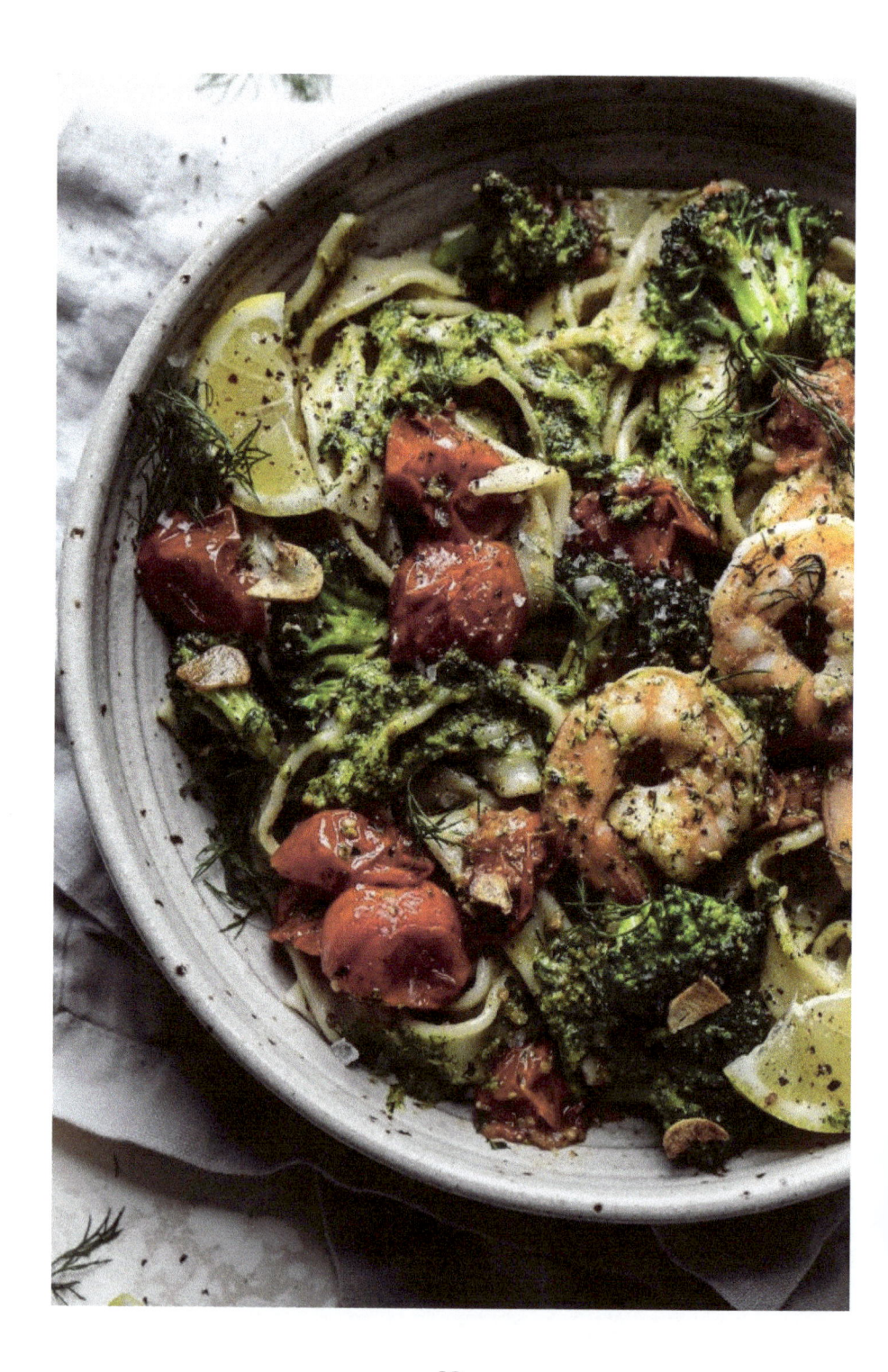

Healthy Apple-licious Chips

Servings per Recipe: 1

Cooking Time: 6 minutes

Ingredients:

- ½ teaspoon ground cumin /2.5G
- 1 apple, cored and sliced thinly
- 1 tablespoon sugar /15G
- A pinch of salt

Instructions:

1) Place all ingredients in a bowl, mix to coat.
2) Put the grill pan in the air fryer and put the sliced apples on the grill pan.
3) Close the air fryer and cook for 6 minutes at 390° F or 199°C.

Nutrition information:

- Calories per serving:130
- Carbs: 33.6g
- Protein: 0.6g
- Fat: 0.5g

Healthy Breakfast Casserole

Servings per Recipe: 2

Cooking Time: 30 minutes

Ingredients:

- ½ cup cooked quinoa /65G
- ½ cup diced bell pepper /65G
- ½ cup shiitake mushrooms, diced /65G
- ½ tsp black pepper /2.5G
- ½ tsp dill /2.5G
- ½ tsp ground cumin /2.5G
- ·½ tsp red pepper flakes /2.5G
- ½ tsp salt /2.5G
- 1 large carrot, peeled and chopped
- 1 small onion, diced
- 1 tbsp lemon juice /15ML
- 1 tsp dried oregano /5G
- 1 tsp garlic, minced /5G
- 1 tsp extra virgin olive oil /5ML
- 2 small celery stalks, chopped
- 2 tbsp soy yogurt, plain /30ML
- 2 tbsp water /30ML
- 2 tbsp yeast /30G
- 7-oz extra firm tofu, drained /210G

Instructions:

1) Grease baking pan with organic olive oil. Add garlic and onion.
2) For 2 minutes, cook at 390° F or 199°C.
3) Remove basket, add bell pepper, celery, and carrots and stir. Cook for 3 minutes.
4) Remove basket, stir in cumin, red pepper flakes, dill, pepper, salt, oregano, and mushrooms. Mix well. Cook for 5 minutes. Mix halfway through cooking time.
5) Blend fresh lemon juice, water, yogurt, yeast, and tofu until creamy.
6) Transfer creamy tofu mixture into air fryer basket. Add quinoa and stir.
7) Cook for an additional 15 minutes at 330° F or 166°C or until golden brown.
8) Allow to cool for 5 minutes.
9) Serve and enjoy.

Nutrition Information:

- Calories per Serving: 280
- Carbs: 28.6g
- Protein: 18.5g
- Fat: 10.1g

Herby Veggie Cornish Pasties

Serves: 4

Cooking Time: 30 Minutes

Ingredients:

- ¼ cup mushrooms, chopped /32.5G
- ¾ cup cold coconut oil /188ML
- 1 ½ cups plain flour /195G
- 1 medium carrot, chopped
- 1 medium potato, diced
- 1 onion, sliced
- 1 stick celery, chopped
- 1 tablespoon nutritional yeast /15G
- 1 tablespoon organic olive oil /15ML
- 1 teaspoon oregano /5G
- a pinch of salt
- cold water for mixing the dough
- salt and pepper to taste

Instructions:

1) Preheat air fryer to 400° F or 205°C.
2) Mix the flour, coconut oil, and salt inside a bowl. Use a fork to combine and gradually add drops of water, stir until you achieve a stiff consistency. Cover the dough with cling film and place in a fridge for 30 minutes.

3) Roll the dough on a flat surface and cut it into squares. Set aside.
4) Heat essential olive oil over medium heat and sauté the onions for two minutes. Add the celery, carrots and potatoes. Continue stirring for 3-5 minutes before adding the mushrooms and oregano.
5) Season with salt and pepper to taste. Add nutritional yeast last. Let it cool as well and set aside.
6) Drop a tablespoon of vegetable mixture onto the dough and seal the sides of the dough with water.
7) Place in the air fryer basket and cook for 20 minutes or when the dough is crispy.

Nutrition information:
- Calories per serving: 659
- Carbohydrates: 56.66g
- Protein: 8.55g
- Fat: 44.97g

Herby Zucchini 'n Eggplant Bake

Serves: 4

Cooking Time: 25 minutes

Ingredients:

- ½ lemon, juiced
- 1 fennel bulb, sliced crosswise
- ·1 sprig flat-leaf parsley
- 1 sprig mint
- 1 sprig of basil
- 1 tablespoon coriander powder /15G
- 1 teaspoon capers /5G
- 2 eggplants, sliced crosswise
- 2 red onions, chopped
- 2 red peppers, sliced crosswise
- 2 teaspoons herb de Provence /10G
- 3 large zucchinis, sliced crosswise
- 4 cloves of garlic, minced
- 4 large tomatoes, chopped
- 5 tablespoons essential olive oil /75ML
- salt and pepper to taste

Instructions:

1) Add basil, parsley, mint, coriander, capers and lemon juice in a blender. Season with salt and pepper to taste. Blend until well combined.
2) Preheat the air fryer to 400° F or 205°C.
3) Place the eggplant, onions, garlic, peppers, fennel, and zucchini with extra virgin olive oil.
4) Arrange the vegetables in a baking pan and pour the tomatoes and also the herb puree. Season with salt and pepper and sprinkle with herbs de Provence.
5) Place inside the air fryer and cook for 25 minutes.

Nutrition information:

- Calories per serving: 375
- Carbohydrates: 47.83g
- Protein: 8.99g
- Fat: 20.03g

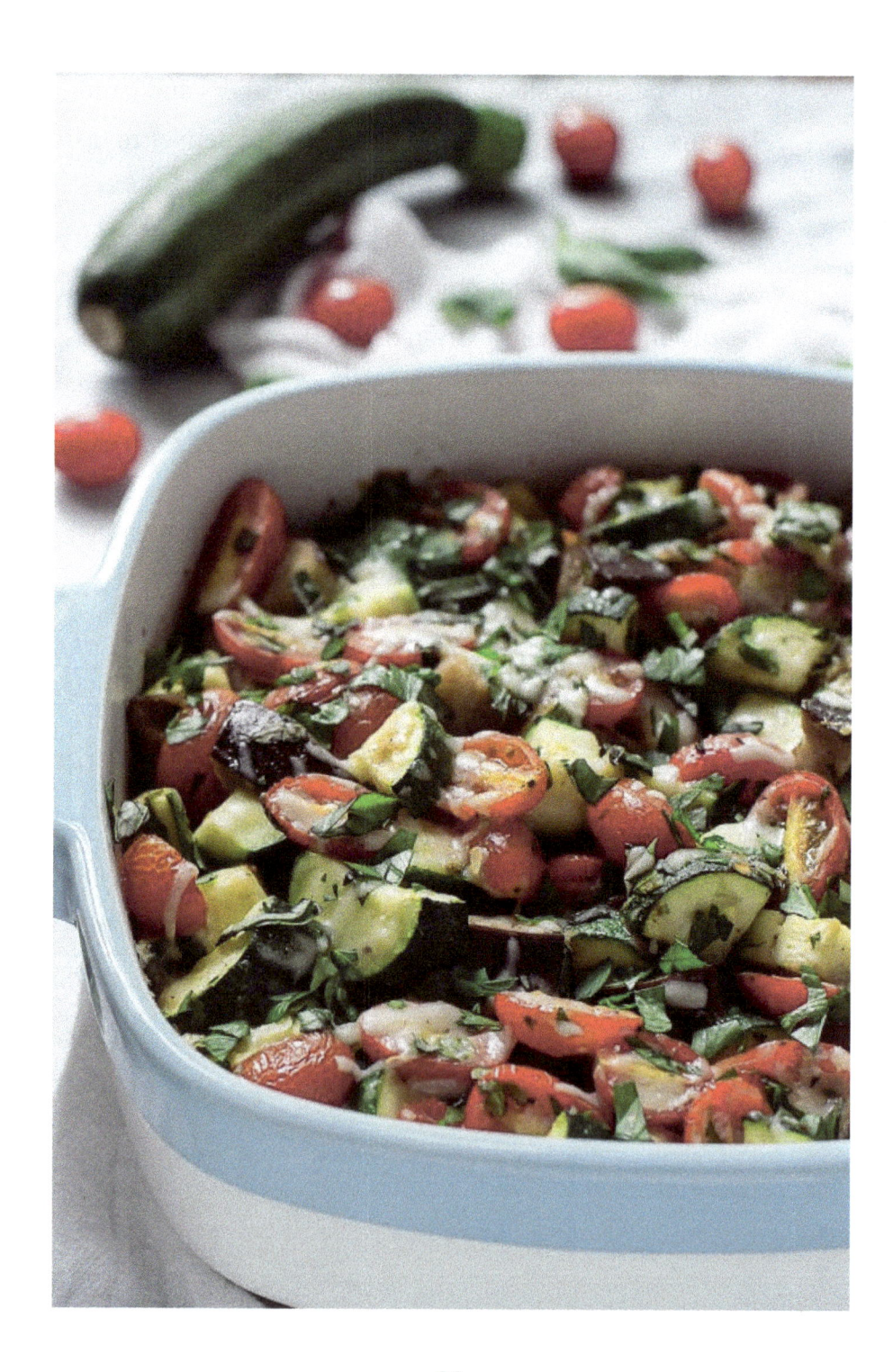

Hollandaise Topped Grilled Asparagus

Servings per Recipe: 6

Cooking Time: 15 minutes

Ingredients:

- ¼ teaspoon black pepper /1.25G
- ½ cup butter, melted /125ML
- ½ lemon juice
- ½ teaspoon salt /2.5G
- ½ teaspoon salt /2.5G
- 1 teaspoon chopped tarragon leaves /2.5G
- 2 tablespoons essential olive oil /30ML
- 3 egg yolks
- 3 pounds asparagus spears, trimmed /1350G
- A pinch of mustard powder
- A punch of ground white pepper

Instructions:

1) Preheat the air fryer to 330° F or 166°C.
2) Place the grill pan in the air fryer.
3) Mix the asparagus, essential olive oil, salt and pepper in a Ziploc bag and shake properly.
4) Place on the grill pan and cook for 15 minutes.

5) Place the double boiler over medium heat, whisk the egg yolks, squeezed fresh lemon juice, and salt until silky. Add the mustard powder, white pepper and melted butter. Keep whisking until the sauce is smooth. Garnish with tarragon leaves.
6) Sprinkle the sauce over asparagus spears.

Nutrition information:

- Calories per serving: 253
- Carbs: 10.2g
- Protein: 6.7g
- Fat: 22.4g

Italian Seasoned Easy Pasta Chips

Servings per Recipe: 2

Cooking Time: 10

Ingredients:

- ½ teaspoon salt /2.5G
- 1 ½ teaspoon Italian seasoning blend /7.5G
- 1 tablespoon nutritional yeast /15G
- 1 tablespoon extra virgin olive oil /15ML
- 2 cups whole wheat bowtie pasta /260G

Instructions

1) Place the baking dish in a mid-air fryer.
2) Stir all the ingredients together and place them in the baking dish.
3) Close mid-air fryer and cook for 10 minutes at 390° F or 199°C .

Nutrition information:

- Calories per serving: 407
- Carbs: 47g
- Protein: 17.9g
- Fat: 17.4g

Jackfruit-Cream Cheese Rangoon

Servings per Recipe: 2

Cooking Time: 10 minutes

Ingredients:

- ¾ Thai curry paste /188ML
- 1 can green jackfruit in brine
- 1 cup vegan cream cheese /130G
- 1 scallion, chopped
- 2 cups vegetable broth /500ML
- 2 teaspoon sesame oil /10ML
- Salt and pepper to taste

Instructions:

1) Place the baking pan in the air fryer.
2) Add the rest of the ingredients and stir well.
3) Close the air fryer and cook for 10 minutes at 390° F or 199°C.

Nutrition information:

- Calories per serving: 457
- Carbs: 107.3g
- Protein: 0.8g
- Fat: 6.8g

Jalapeno Stuffed with Bacon 'n Cheeses

Serves: 8

Cooking Time: 15 minutes

Ingredients:

- ¼ cup cheddar cheese, shredded /32.5G
- 1 teaspoon paprika /5G
- 16 fresh jalapenos, sliced lengthwise and seeded
- 16 strips of uncured bacon, cut into half
- 4-ounce cream cheese /120G
- Salt to taste

Instructions:

1) Mix the cream cheese, cheddar cheese, salt, and paprika in a bowl until well-combined.
2) Put half a teaspoon onto each half of jalapeno peppers.
3) Wrap a thin strip of bacon across the cheese-filled jalapeno half. Put on gloves when doing this because jalapeno is quite spicy.
4) Place in mid-air fryer basket and cook for 15 minutes in a 350° F or 177°C preheated air fryer.

Nutrition information:

- Calories per serving: 225
- Carbohydrates: 3.2g

- Protein: 10.6g
- Fat: 18.9g

Layered Tortilla Bake

Servings per Recipe: 6

Cooking Time: 30 Minutes

Ingredients:

- 1 (15 ounces) can black beans, rinsed and drained /450G
- 1 cup salsa /130G
- 1 cup salsa, divided /130G
- 1/2 cup chopped tomatoes /65G
- 1/2 cup sour cream /125ML
- 2 (15 ounces) cans pinto beans, drained and rinsed /450G
- 2 cloves garlic, minced
- 2 cups shredded reduced-fat Cheddar cheese /260G
- 2 tablespoons chopped fresh cilantro /30G
- 7 (8 inches) flour tortillas

Instructions:

1) Mash pinto beans in a large bowl and mix in garlic and salsa.
2) Mix tomatoes, black beans, cilantro, and ¼ cup salsa in a bowl.

3) Grease baking pan of air fryer with cooking spray. Spread 1 tortilla, spread ¾ cup pinto bean mixture evenly approximately ½-inch away from the edge of tortilla, spread ¼ cup cheese ahead. Cover with another tortilla spread 2/3 cup black bean mixture after which ¼ cup cheese. Repeat the layering. Cover with the last tortilla, top with pinto bean mixture then cheese.
4) Cover the pan with foil.
5) Cook for 25 minutes at 390° F or 199°C , remove foil and cook for 5 minutes or until tops are lightly browned.
6) Serve and get.

Nutrition Information:

- Calories per Serving: 409
- Carbs: 54.8g
- Protein: 21.1g
- Fat: 11.7g

Loaded Brekky Hash Browns

Servings per Recipe: 4

Cooking Time: 20 Minutes

Ingredients:

- 3 russet potatoes, peeled and grated
- 2 garlic cloves chopped
- 1 teaspoon paprika /5G
- salt and pepper to taste
- 1 teaspoon canola oil /5ML
- 1 teaspoon olive oil /5ML
- 1/4 cup chopped green peppers /32.5
- 1/4 cup chopped red peppers /32.5G
- 1/4 cup chopped onions /32.5G

Instructions:

1) Soak the grated potatoes for 20 minutes in a bowl of cold water. Drain and dry with paper towels.
2) Grease baking pan of air fryer with cooking spray.
3) Add grated potatoes to the air fryer. Season with garlic, paprika, salt, and pepper. Add canola and organic olive oil. Mix well to coat.
4) Cook on 390° F or 199°C for 10 minutes.
5) Remove the basket and place the ball mixture in it. Add green, red peppers, onions and stir.

6) Cook for another 10 minutes.
7) Serve and enjoy.

Nutrition Information:

- Calories per Serving: 263
- Carbs: 53.2g
- Protein: 6.5g
- Fat: 2.6g

Melted Cheese 'n Almonds on Tomato

Servings per Recipe: 3

Cooking Time: 20 minutes

Ingredients:

- ¼ cup toasted almonds /32.5G
- 1 yellow red bell pepper, chopped
- 3 large tomatoes
- 4 ounces Monterey Jack cheese /120G
- Salt and pepper to taste

Instructions:

1) Preheat air fryer to 330° F or 166°C.
2) Place the grill pan in the air fryer.
3) Slice off the tops of the tomatoes and remove the seeds to make hollow "cups."
4) Add the cheese, bell pepper, and almonds to a mixing bowl. Season with salt and pepper to taste.
5) Stuff the tomatoes with the cheese filling.
6) Place the stuffed tomatoes in the grill pan and cook for 15 to 20 minutes.

Nutrition information:

- Calories per serving: 125
- Carbs: 13g

- Protein: 10g
- Fat: 14g

Minty Green Beans with Shallots

Servings per Recipe: 6

Cooking Time: 25 minutes

Ingredients:

- 1 tablespoon fresh mint, chopped /15G
- 1 tablespoon sesame seeds, toasted /15G
- 1 tablespoon vegetable oil /15ML
- 1 teaspoon soy sauce /5ML
- 1-pound fresh green beans, trimmed /450G
- 2 large shallots, sliced
- 2 tablespoons fresh basil, chopped /30G
- 2 tablespoons pine nuts /30G

Instructions:

1) Preheat air fryer to 330° F or 166°C.
2) Place the grill pan in the air fryer.
3) Add the green beans, shallots, vegetable oil, and soy sauce to a mixing bowl.
4) Place in the air fryer and cook for 25 minutes.
5) Once cooked, garnish with basil, mints, sesame seeds, and pine nuts.

Nutrition information:

- Calories per serving: 307

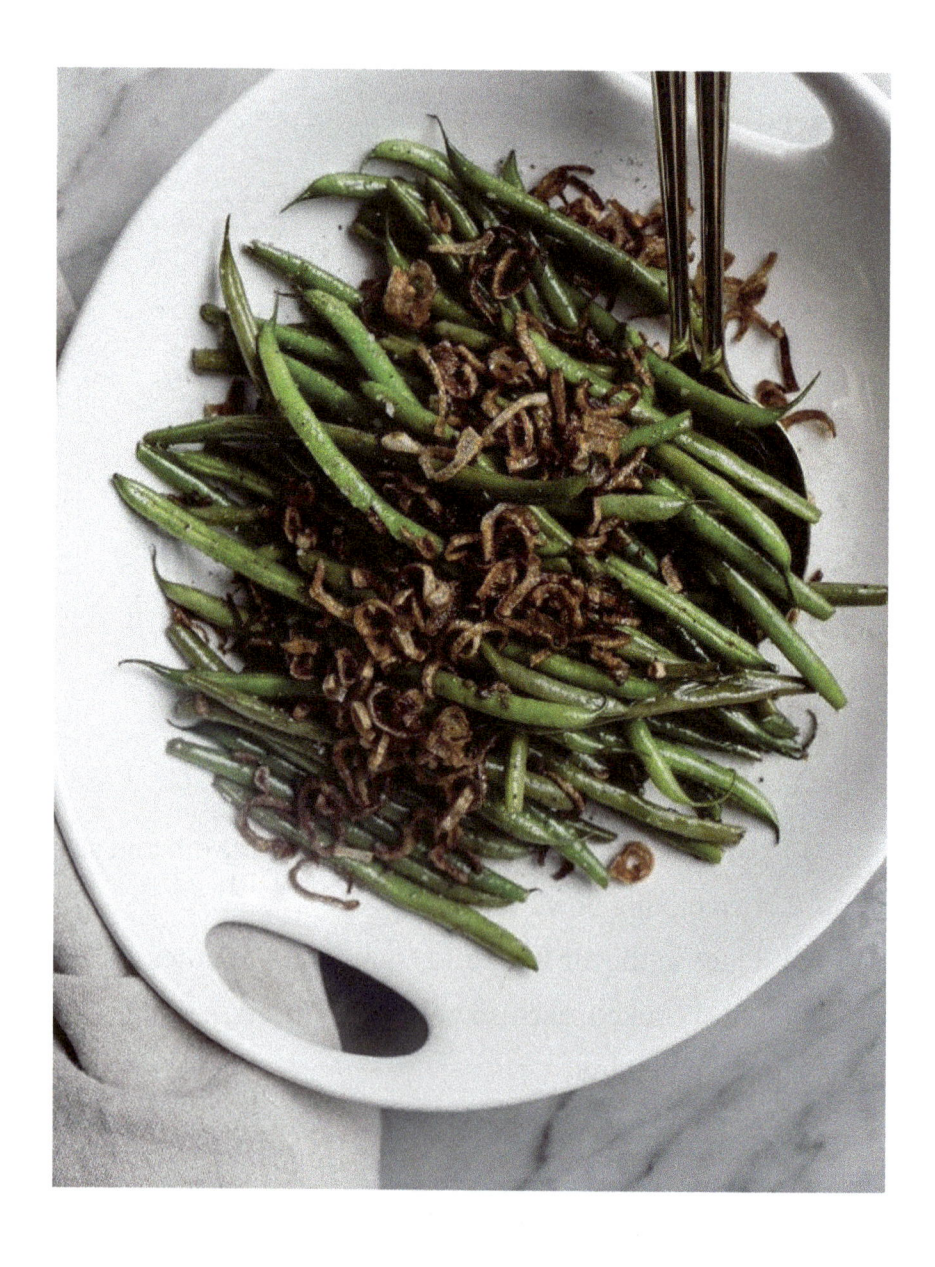

- Carbs: 11.2g
- Protein: 23.7g
- Fat: 19.7g